Clinical Applications of the Therapeutic Powers of Play

Clinical Applications of the Therapeutic Powers of Play provides a way to link abstract theory with practice-based knowledge and vice versa, navigating the complexities of clinical reasoning associated with age-sensitive and most often non-verbal psychotherapies.

The book invites readers into the world of child psychotherapy and into the play therapy room. It equips them to explore, discover and identify the therapeutic powers of play in action, within traditional and nature-based therapeutic environments. Using embodiment-projective-role, it navigates the developmental stages linking play and the achievement of physical, emotional and social identity. With captivating stories of hope and repair, the book deconstructs the therapy process to better understand how play facilitates communication, fosters emotional wellness, increases personal strengths and enhances social relationships.

This comprehensive text will help the therapist navigate through the world of child and adolescent psychotherapy and explain the therapeutic powers of play through relevant clinical case studies.

Eileen Prendiville is the Director of Academic Affairs at the Children's Therapy Centre (CTC) in Westmeath, Ireland. She founded this centre and designed its play therapy and psychotherapy training programmes including the Master of Arts in Creative Psychotherapy. She was also a founding member of the Children at Risk in Ireland Foundation and was National Clinical Director until 2004 when she moved to CTC.

Judi A. Parson Ph.D., MA Play Therapy, M.Hth Sc., G.Dip Paeds, RN, RPT-S (APPTA and BAPT). Academic Course Director, Master of Child Play Therapy, Deakin University. Judi supervises a range of play therapy research projects and Ph.D. students and maintains a small private practice.

Clinical Applications of the Therapeutic Powers of Play

Case Studies in Child and Adolescent Psychotherapy

Edited by Eileen Prendiville
and Judi A. Parson

Routledge
Taylor & Francis Group

LONDON AND NEW YORK

First published 2021
by Routledge
2 Park Square, Milton Park, Abingdon, Oxon OX14 4RN

and by Routledge
52 Vanderbilt Avenue, New York, NY 10017

Routledge is an imprint of the Taylor & Francis Group, an informa business

British Library Cataloguing-in-Publication Data
A catalogue record for this book is available from the British Library

Library of Congress Cataloging-in-Publication Data
A catalog record has been requested for this book

ISBN: 978-0-367-34108-4 (hbk)
ISBN: 978-0-367-34109-1 (pbk)
ISBN: 978-0-429-32394-2 (ebk)

Typeset in Sabon
by MPS Limited, Dehradun

Dedications

Play – always and forever! Before there were grandchildren there were children … and before there were children there was a couple … and before that there were siblings and parents. Much love to all my family, every one of you has brought love, joy and playfulness into my life.

Let the fun continue!

Eileen

I would like to dedicate this book to my parents, Kathleen and David Parson, who have always supported me in achieving my dreams.

Thank you!

Judi 'Ali' Parson

In memory of our mentor and dear friend:

Dr Charles E. Schaefer

1933–2020

A curious, playful sort of wise wizard who took delight in questions and taught us to apply the therapeutic powers of play. May his legacy live on in the lives of all children healed through play therapy.

Rest In Peace Charlie

Eileen and Judi

Contents

Figures and Tables

Figures

Tables

Editors

Eileen Prendiville is the Director of Academic Affairs and a core trainer for the MA in Creative Psychotherapy (Humanistic & Integrative Modality), and the Postgraduate Diploma in Play Therapy, at the Children's Therapy Centre in Co Westmeath, Ireland. Eileen was a founder member, and National Clinical Director, of the Children at Risk in Ireland Foundation, Ireland's specialist treatment service for children and families affected by child sexual abuse. Eileen is a psychotherapist, play therapist, supervisor and trainer. Eileen co-edited *Play Therapy Today: Contemporary practice with individuals, groups, and carers* and *Creative Psychotherapy: Applying the principles of neurobiology to play and expressive arts-based practice* published by Routledge. She has written many book chapters. She is strongly involved in Ireland's professional associations (the Irish Association of Humanistic & Integrative Psychotherapy and the Irish Association for Play Therapy and Psychotherapy) governing play therapy and psychotherapy in Ireland. Eileen devised 'The Therapeutic Touchstone', an innovative approach for use when working with vulnerable and dependent clients.

Judi A. Parson, Ph.D., MA Play Therapy, RN, BN. is a qualified paediatric Registered Nurse, Play Therapist, Senior Lecturer in Play Therapy and Disipline Leader and Course Director for the Therapeutic Play and Child Play Therapy courses at Deakin University, Australia. Judi is a Registered Play Therapist and Supervisor with the Australasia Pacific Play Therapy Association (APPTA) and the British Association of Play Therapists (BAPT). Judi, a founding director and past Chair of APPTA, continues as an active board member. She also sits on the Advisory Board for the International Centre for Children and Family Law Inc (ICCFL). The focus of her research is based on the establishment of evidence to understand how to best serve at risk populations, such as children who are vulnerable due to play deficits, ethnicity, health status and/or socioeconomic situation. She has a special interest in working with children who have experienced medical trauma and life-limiting illnesses. Judi has authored over 15 internationally peer-reviewed journal articles and book chapters, and she is often invited to provide keynote presentations throughout Australia, Asia and the UK.

Contributors

Sue C. Bratton, Ph.D., LPC-S, RPT-S, is Professor Emeritus in the Counseling Program and Director Emeritus, Center for Play Therapy, at the University of North Texas, with over 30 years of experience as a practitioner and researcher. Sue is an internationally known speaker and author with over 90 publications and 300 professional presentations in the areas of play therapy and child and family counseling with a specific focus on research examining the effectiveness of child-centred play therapy and child-parent relationship therapy. She is co-author of *Child Parent Relationship Therapy (CPRT)*, the *CPRT Treatment Manual, CPRT in Action, Child-Centered Play Therapy Research,* and *Integrative Play Therapy*. Sue is a Past President and board member of the Association for Play Therapy (APT). She is also recipient of many awards including the APT Lifetime Achievement Award, APT Outstanding Research Award, American Counseling Association (ACA) Extended Research Award, ACA Best Practice Award, American Humanistic Counseling Educator/Supervisor Award and Chi Sigma Iota Outstanding Practitioner Supervisor Award. She is an active social advocate for children at the local, national and international level, particularly underserved children who have faced traumatic life experiences.

Athena A. Drewes, PsyD, MA, RPT-S, is a licensed Psychologist and Registered Play Therapist-Supervisor. She is former Director of Clinical Training and APA-Accredited Doctoral Internship at Astor Services for Children and Families, a large multi-service non-profit mental health agency in New York. She has over 45 years of clinical experience in supervision and clinical work with complex trauma, sexually abused, traumatised and attachment-disordered children and adolescents in school, outpatient, foster care and inpatient settings. She is a former Board Director of the Association for Play Therapy and Founder and President Emeritus of the New York Association for Play Therapy. She has written extensively on play therapy and is an invited guest lecturer in the US, Taiwan, England, Ireland, Argentina, Mexico, Denmark, Canada and Italy. She has edited/co-edited 12 books including *The Therapeutic Powers of Play: 20 Core Agents of Change, Puppet Play Therapy* and *Play Therapy in Middle Childhood*. This latter book, published by the American Psychological Association, has a companion video DVD of Dr. Drewes' integrative prescriptive play therapy work.

Carol Duffy holds an MA in Creative Psychotherapy (Humanistic and Integrative Modality), a professional Diploma in Child Psychotherapy and Play Therapy, and a Diploma in Creative Supervision. She is an accredited child and adolescent psychotherapist who specialises in play therapy. Carol has been working with children for close to 20 years and is employed as a senior play therapist working with children and young people. Her work is also strongly influenced by neurobiological and attachment perspectives, with an emphasis on sensory integration and regulation. She offers substantial support to the family and care systems of her primary clients. Carol has significant experience of working with children in care and with children who have experienced attachment disruptions and developmental/relational trauma. Carol is a core trainer on the MA programme in the Children's Therapy Centre, in Westmeath, Ireland, and has a private practice where she offers creative supervision. Carol has completed research on the use of regulating and relational play skills in social work practice to enhance social worker-child relationships and developed a model called the R.R.I.G.H.T. Play Therapy Techniques.

Maggie Fearn, SFHEA, MA HIPPT, MA DAPT, BAPT, is a Senior Lecturer in Play Therapy and Therapeutic Studies at the University of South Wales; visiting lecturer with the Children's Therapy Centre, Ireland; and child and adolescent psychotherapist, play therapist, filial therapist and clinical supervisor with The Windfall Centre in Wales. She regularly contributes articles and chapters on a range of topics related to relational play as a medium for therapeutic growth, and she is internationally recognised for her contributions to nature-based play therapy theory and practice.

Ken Gardner, M.Sc., R. Psych (CPT-S), is a Clinical Psychologist and certified play therapy supervisor with over 25 years of counseling experience. Through the Rocky Mountain Play Therapy Institute, Ken has presented nationally and internationally on a wide range of topics related to play therapy and supervision. Ken has served as an executive board member on the Canadian Association for Play Therapy. His specialisations include play-based interventions for children with developmental challenges. Ken has written several chapters on play therapy and is the co-editor of *Turning Points in Play Therapy and the*

Emergence of Self: Applications of the Play Therapy Dimensions Model (2019), and co-author of *The Play Therapy Dimensions Model: A Decision-Making Guide for Integrative Play Therapists* (2012).

Paris Goodyear-Brown, LCSW, RPT-S, is the Clinical Director of Nurture House, the Executive Director of the TraumaPlay™ Institute and the creator of TraumaPlay™, a flexibly sequential play therapy model for treating childhood trauma. She is an internationally sought after teacher, a master clinician, an EMDRIA Certified therapist and a TBRI Educator with 25 years of experience in treating traumatised and attachment disturbed children and families. She is an Adjunct Instructor of Psychiatric Mental Health at Vanderbilt University, gave a TedTalk and trains therapists, parents and teachers around the globe. She has received the APT award for Play Therapy Promotion and Education and is the author of multiple books, chapters and articles related to child therapy. Her most recent books include *Parents as Partners in Child Therapy: A Clinician's Guide* and *Trauma and Play Therapy: Helping Children Heal.*

Henry Kronengold, Ph.D., maintains a private psychotherapy practice in New York City. He is a clinical supervisor at the Clinical Psychology Program at the City University of New York. His book, *Stories from Child & Adolescent Psychotherapy*, explores the unpredictable world of child and adolescent psychotherapy through a series of engaging and innovative clinical vignettes.

Siobhán Prendiville, MA in Humanistic and Integrative Psychotherapy and Play Therapy, M.Ed, B.Ed, is Course Leader for the MA in Creative Psychotherapy (Humanistic & Integrative Modality), which incorporates a Postgraduate Diploma in Play Therapy, at the Children's Therapy Centre (CTC) in Ireland. CTC is the longest established and foremost provider of professional play therapy training in Ireland. It is currently the only institution in Ireland where students can gain a dual qualification as a Play Therapist and Psychotherapist with full academic and professional validation. Siobhán is a child and adolescent psychotherapist, play therapist, clinical supervisor, author, presenter and trainer. She also maintains a private child and adolescent psychotherapy and play therapy practice. Siobhán is fully accredited with the Irish Association for Play Therapy and Psychotherapy and with the Irish Association of Humanistic & Integrative Psychotherapy. She has published many chapters in the play therapy domain.

Kate Renshaw, B. Psych, Grad. Grad. Dip. Art Therapy, Dip. Play Therapy and, Ph.D. Candidate, is a Play and Filial Therapist and an academic at Deakin University. As a Lecturer in Play Therapy she is responsible for providing education, research and supervision in Play Therapy, and teaches the Graduate Certificate/Diploma of Therapeutic Child Play and Master of Child Play Therapy. Kate is a Registered Play Therapist with the British Association of Play Therapists (BAPT) and an RPT-S with the Australasia Pacific Play Therapy Association (APPTA). Kate is currently completing doctoral studies investigating the development and efficacy of the Teacher's Optimal Relationship Approach (TORA), which integrates play and filial therapy principles into the education setting. In her private practice, she works therapeutically with children and families as well as offering clinical supervision to Play Therapists Australia wide. Kate has been a member of the Board of Directors for APPTA since 2013.

Karen Stagnitti, OT, Ph.D., was Professor, Personal Chair at the School of Health and Social Development at Deakin University, Geelong, Australia, until retirement in December 2018. She is now Emeritus Professor in the School of Health and Social Development at Deakin University, Geelong, Australia. Over the past 40 years she has worked in early childhood intervention programs in community-based settings as part of specialist paediatric multidisciplinary teams and as a research and teaching academic. In 2003 she graduated from LaTrobe University with a Doctor of Philosophy. Her area of research is children's play. Karen has over 120 publications including national and international papers peer-reviewed journal articles, books and book chapters. Her norm referenced standardised play assessment, the Child-Initiated Pretend Play Assessment-2, has been used in several research studies examining relationships between pretend play, language and social skills; social-emotional understanding and play complexity; play ability in children with autism spectrum disorder and abilities of children who attend different types of school curriculum. She developed learn to play therapy for children with developmental difficulties who do not have play skills. This therapy approach is now used in several countries.

Alyssa M. Swan, Ph.D., LCPC, RPT, NCC, Certified CCPT-S, Certified CPRT-S, is an Assistant Professor and the Training Director in the Ph.D. Counselor Education program at Adler University in Chicago, IL. Dr. Swan served as a Robert B. Toulouse Research Fellow and Assistant Director at the Center for Play Therapy at the University of North Texas for over three years. She is a graduate of the Association for Play Therapy Leadership Academy and received the Dissertation Research Award from the Association for Play Therapy in 2018. Dr. Swan served as the Associate Clinical Director at the Children's Home of Poughkeepsie in Poughkeepsie, NY in 2019.

Lorri Yasenik, Ph.D., MSW, RPT-S, CPT-S, is a Co-Director of Rocky Mountain Play Therapy Institute in Calgary Alberta, Canada. Lorri is the co-author of the *Play Therapy Dimensions Model: A Decision-*

Making Model for Integrative Play Therapists (2012) and *Turning Points in Play Therapy and the Emergence of Self: Applications of the Play Therapy Dimensions Model* (2019) as well as many book chapters on play therapy supervision and play therapy techniques. Lorri is a certified and registered play therapist supervisor and a founding member of Alberta Play Therapy Association. She trains nationally and internationally in the areas of play therapy, child psychotherapy, attachment, trauma and high conflict separation and divorce.

Foreword

Judi A. Parson and Eileen Prendiville

It all began in 2018 at the International Play Therapy Study Group (IPTSG). This is an annual event where a small group of play therapists were personally invited by Dr Charles Schaefer to come together and share knowledge, joy and laughter while engaging in fascinating discussions at the forefront of our field. The authors identified what we saw as a significant gap in available literature and excitedly decided to address it. We wanted to bring the therapeutic powers of play (TPoP) to life by highlighting their transformative powers in actual case studies, and to overlay this with Jennings' (1999) embodiment-projection-role (EPR) model to examine how the three play categories support the development of physical, emotional and social identity and contextualise the process of therapy in action. And so this book was conceived.

When we excitedly discussed the idea of co-editing this book, we could visualise using the metaphorical images of landscapes, continents and the four corners of the world to provide the organisational backdrop to explore the scope and scale of how play enhances and facilitates therapeutic change in clinical practice. We are well positioned, after all we are geographically located about 17,375 km apart, so it made sense that we needed to embark on this project from a global perspective. So, from either side of the world we believed we could provide a solid mark in the landscape to help the therapist navigate through the therapeutic powers of play within the theory-practice discourse. The following provides an orientation to the structure of this book and each section includes four unique chapters.

Section 1: The Landscape

The first section of this book sets the scene and focusses on the landscape by presenting a baseline summary of who, what, why, when and where the therapeutic powers of play emerged and how they may be theoretically and practically integrated in order to understand and map change along the therapeutic process. The first chapter introduces the TPoP as the 20 core agents of change (Schaefer & Drewes, 2014). Prendiville follows by presenting, exploring and expanding on Jennings' (1999) developmental EPR paradigm in order to inform the child and adolescent psychotherapist

(Chapter 2). These two core positions then scaffold the reader to consider the scope and scale of how play enhances and facilitates therapeutic change in clinical practice. Importantly both perspectives provide a different viewpoint to examine the TPoP and play development without the need to rely on any one particular theoretical model of practice but rather both provide a lens in which to track therapeutic change. Goodyear-Brown (Chapter 3) provides an overview of traditional play therapy settings and presents a rich discussion and accompanying images of developmentally sensitive clinical play therapy spaces and ideas in order to apply the therapeutic powers of play in practice. To finalise the landscape setting, Fearn (Chapter 4) takes the reader from the indoors to the outdoors and into nature using a case study to demonstrate the healing power of nature play.

Section 2: Travelling through the continents

In order to facilitate transformative thinking, we reasoned that presenting relevant clinical case studies, signposting the developmental stages would help to reveal and explore the specific therapeutic powers of play along the EPR sequence. Siobhan Prendiville (Chapter 5) commences this section with the embodiment stage and skilfully weaves sensory play activities within an integrative framework to showcase examples from the clinical world where all 20 agents of change were activated. Through sensory play Christopher finds joy and a happier and healthier way of being. The next developmental step, projective play, presented by Renshaw and Parson (Chapter 6) brings together evidence from the literature, integrative humanistic play therapy and the therapeutic powers of small world play and links theory with clinical practice through Amber's story. Furthermore, Stagnitti (Chapter 7) expertly brings together the art and science of pretence whereby Jonathon, a five-year-old boy with autism, learns to play. Then Duffy (Chapter 8) concludes the EPR sequence and presents early life developmental trauma with specific reference to the therapeutic role play journey of Sally. Together the chapters bring to life the specific therapeutic powers of play according to the developmental stage.

Section 4: Connecting the four corners of the world

In this section the four corners of the world provide the metaphorical backdrop to represent the four major categories of the therapeutic powers of play. Each of the chapters explore in greater detail and link clinical cases in how play facilitates communication, fosters emotional wellness, increases personal strengths and enhances social relationships. Swan and Bratton (Chapter 9) present a clinical case of Alex, who has a reactive attachment disorder (RAD), and identifies powers including self-expression, access to the unconscious, direct teaching and indirect teaching. Yasenik (Chapter 10) identifies many TPoP (catharsis, abreaction, positive emotion, counterconditioning fears, stress inoculation and stress management) through the magic of Polly the puppet who meets three-and-a-half-year-old Maddie, and facilitates her in disclosing, and processing, trauma. In the next (Chapter 11) Gardner presents two case studies with Bradley and then Sammy and the three-legged cat to demonstrate how a contextual and developmentally sensitive approach must be taken when examining therapeutic relationship, attachment, social competence and empathy. Kronengold (Chapter 12) takes us on a fast-paced race to Le Mans to demonstrate how Danny increased his personal strength and resiliency. The therapeutic powers activated in this category include creative problem solving, resiliency, moral development, accelerated psychological development, self-regulation and self-esteem.

All developmentally appropriate models of child psychotherapy share one common feature – the use of play. Regardless of the theory of change on which the therapist relies, play itself is the enzyme that aids the digestion of unresolved material and overwhelming emotions. Understanding how these enzymes work, and may be applied, has relevance for all practitioners working in diverse contexts with children and adolescents. In this book we look at play through the lens of a developmental paradigm, exploring play that is linked to physical, emotional and social identity.

Finally, in the conclusion, Drewes draws together the manuscript as a whole to a close by highlighting the pertinent and concluding ideas and concepts identified throughout each of the three sections. This book provides a way to link abstract theory with practice-based knowledge and vice versa, thus navigating the complexities of clinical reasoning associated with age-sensitive, developmentally appropriate and most often non-verbal psychotherapies.

References

Jennings, S. (1999). *An introduction to developmental playtherapy*. London: Jessica Kingsley.

Schaefer, C. E., & Drewes A. A. (2014). *The therapeutic powers of play: 20 core agents of change*. (2nd ed.). Hoboken, NJ: John Wiley.

Part I

The landscape

You are invited to travel into the world of child psychotherapy and right into the play therapy room. An embodiment-projective-role lens is provided to equip you to explore, discover and identify the therapeutic powers of play in action. The landscape includes traditional, clinical and nature-based therapeutic environments.

Chapter 1

Children speak play
Landscaping the therapeutic powers of play

Judi A. Parson

Play is full of contradictions! Eberle (2014, p. 232) states that

> *Play can be challenging or soothing, rough or gentle, physical or intellectual, mischievous or well mannered, orderly or disorderly, competitive or cooperative, planned or spontaneous, solitary or social, inventive or rule-bound, simple or complex, or strenuous or restful ...*

This complexity makes play difficult to define, yet we do know when we see it and we do know when it is absent. Brown (2010) identifies a number of play properties and states that play is fun, it is done for its own sake, it is voluntary, in play there is a lost sense of time, and it feels so good that you want to keep doing it. Eberle (2014) defines play according to six basic elements namely these: anticipation, surprise, pleasure, understanding, strength and poise. Eberle goes on to expand on these elements to identify kindred terms as well as when a play element is no longer play: for example, when anticipation becomes obsession, surprise becomes shock or terror, or understanding becomes indifference and so on (Eberle, 2014). Chazan (2002) and Brown (2010) also differentiate play from pre-play (selecting and setting up toys and play materials), non-play (needing to take a drink or snack, or read the instructions or chatting with the therapist) and play in-terruptions (when the child abruptly stops the play or non-play sequence due to rising tension within the session and may be signalled when the child needs to go to the bathroom or check where their parents are). Play therapists are interested in understanding multiple contexts and aspects within the child's play landscape.

> *Play activity is infinitely variable and is identifiable by the non-verbal attributes of focused concentration, purposeful choice of toy or object and specific affective expression.*
>
> (Chazan, 2002, p. 28)

There are multiple types and descriptions for play including the following: sensory, gross motor, rough and tumble, exploratory, construction, problem solving, pretend, projective, traumatic or abreactive play, role play, games, musical expression, arts and craft activities and nature play. However, within this book a clear developmental alignment is presented through the embodiment-projective-role (EPR) sequence (Jennings, 1999) and incorporates many, if not all, of the play activities mentioned earlier in relation to the therapeutic powers of play landscape.

Play is not secondary to the therapy – it is the therapy

Healing happens through play! The play, in play therapy, is not a trick or lure, or even a warm-up exercise, nor is it a pre-requisite into conversation. It is, however, both the therapeutic medium and the process which promotes growth and development. Just as enzymes produced in the body act as a catalyst to bring about specific biochemical reactions to transfer, change or join molecules within the physical body, the therapeutic powers of play are the enzymes to transfer, change, join and aid in the digestion of emotional material and facilitate movement towards optimal psychosocial and emotional health and well-being. In play children are safe to draw on any number of possibilities, to pretend and process unresolved material, to change the emotional tone of past memories and to allow for the transfer of previously intrusive memories to past memory. In essence, play is the developmentally appropriate medium for children in therapy.

The therapeutic powers of play framework

During the 2017 International Play Therapy Study Group (IPTSG) hosted by Professor Emeritus Charles Schaefer, Fairleigh Dickinson University, I presented on 'Puppets in play therapy'. I used a novel methodical approach called Integrating, Theory, Evidence and Action (ITEA) (Hitch, Pepin, & Stagnitti, 2014) to systemically review the literature. This approach incorporates several steps including the following: creating a clinical question, choosing a suitable framework or model to provide a lens to examine the literature, identifying the search strategy and databases and deconstructing and analysing the extracted data in order to reconstruct and subsequently transfer and utilise the data in a way to give back meaning to clinical practitioners (Hitch et al., 2014). I chose the TPoP as the framework to answer the question 'How does puppet play enhance the therapeutic effect for children (age range 0–18 years) requiring therapy?' But as part of the process to identify the TPoP in action, I developed a graphic (see Figure 1.1) to systematically record and summarise findings in order to quickly extract coded data and calculate which of the major categories and the specific therapeutic powers of play were represented in each paper. While the image

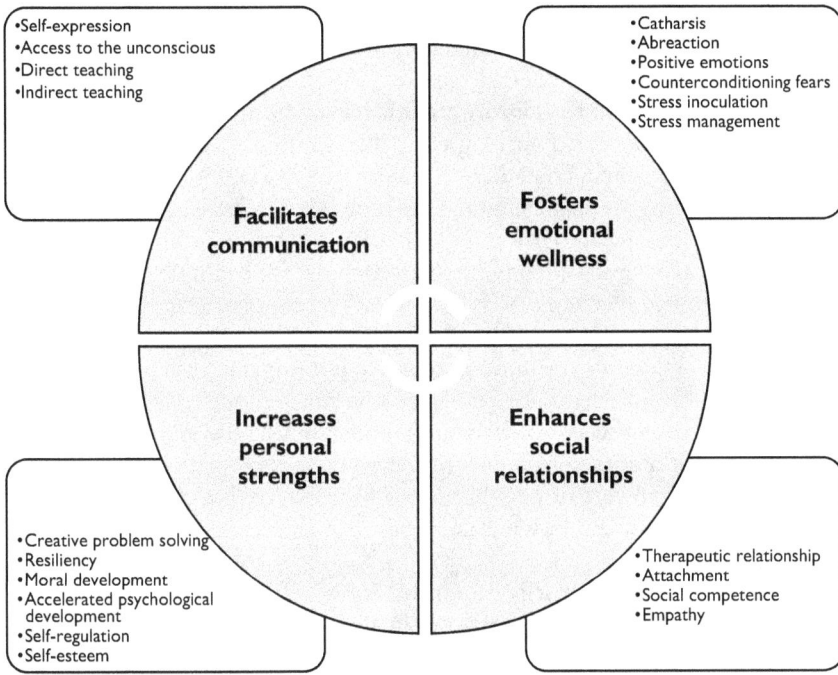

- Self-expression
- Access to the unconscious
- Direct teaching
- Indirect teaching

- Catharsis
- Abreaction
- Positive emotions
- Counterconditioning fears
- Stress inoculation
- Stress management

Facilitates communication

Fosters emotional wellness

Increases personal strengths

Enhances social relationships

- Creative problem solving
- Resiliency
- Moral development
- Accelerated psychological development
- Self-regulation
- Self-esteem

- Therapeutic relationship
- Attachment
- Social competence
- Empathy

Figure 1.1 The therapeutic powers of play: 20 core agents of change.
Note: Graphic created by Judi A. Parson adapted from Schaefer C. E., & Drewes A. A. (2014). The therapeutic powers of play: 20 core agents of change. (2nd ed.). Hoboken, N.J: John Wiley.

presented here is in greyscale, I colour coded the major categories, using neon highlighter pens, pink, yellow, green and orange, to aid the data extraction process of the ITEA. I must acknowledge my colleague Kate Renshaw, who was accurate with the highlighter pen, who validated the coding methodology, and together we reviewed and cross checked all 55 articles.

The IPTSG attendees appreciated the graphic as a simple visual aid that captured the essential therapeutic powers of play at a glance. But what the ITEA did was provide a way to evidence the therapeutic effect (i.e. the change mechanism) as presented in the literature, and while puppet play was the focus of the presentation, the TPoP graphic could be adapted to investigate any phenomena within play therapy literature and/or clinical practice. The beauty of integrating various forms of evidence using the ITEA method provided accessibility to other ways of knowing which could be included to inform the clinical direction and action required based on the specific topic matter or problem. This is a useful method because it is a fundamental necessity for child and adolescent psychotherapists and play therapists to know what, why, how and when the *play* within the clinical intervention produces positive change in the child client. Thus, the TPoP framework provides a powerful lens to examine the literature as well as clinical cases, which in turn informs clinical reasoning and decision making before, during and after the therapeutic intervention.

The TPoP were first coined by Schaefer (1993) when he identified 14 basic mechanisms of change and then later expanded these to 20 core agents (Schaefer, 2020). They may be explained, explored and understood through multiple ways and may be referred to as 'for example, "therapeutic powers," "change mechanisms," "mediators of change," "causal factors," and "principles of therapeutic action"' (Drewes & Schaefer, 2014, p. 1). However, the TPoP may be difficult to grasp initially, because of their trans-theoretical nature: they do not belong to one single model, but, rather, they present an abstract way to view and understand how play acts as the medium to 'initiate, facilitate or strengthen their therapeutic effect' (p. 2). The therapeutic powers of play have also been referred to as 'the heart and soul of play therapy' (p. 4), which signifies that they are essential knowledge to clinical practice.

As a threshold concept it is important for play therapists to understand the TPoP as core knowledge early on in their play therapy education and supervised practice. Meyer and Land (2003, p. 1) state that:

> *A threshold concept can be considered as akin to a portal, opening up a new and previously inaccessible way of thinking about something. It represents a transformed way of understanding, or interpreting, or viewing something without which the learner cannot progress. As a consequence of comprehending a threshold concept there may thus be a transformed internal view of subject matter, subject landscape, or even world view.*

Understanding that threshold concepts are transformative, this book aims to transform the reader's comprehension of the subject matter (clinical applications of the therapeutic powers of play) through the experience and wisdom of internationally distinguished authors who have contributed to this edition. Schaefer and Drewes (2014) presented a list of 20 core agents of change in four distinct categories, namely that play (1) facilitates communication, (2) fosters emotional wellness, (3) increases personal strengths and (4) enhances social relationships (see Figure 1.1). The specific therapeutic powers of play are now briefly summarised and italicised for easy recognition throughout this chapter.

Facilitates communication

Children speak play! Play therapists are educated to speak play too because play is the most developmentally accessible means of communicating with children. Play facilitates *self-expression* because children may not have or do not want to use words when concrete forms of expression provide a more age-appropriate way to convey meaning. For example, children, through selecting and arranging toys in specific ways, drawing a picture of their family or crafting a playdough image of a snake or snail, provide information as subjective content. However, the play therapist may understand the play activity through a range of cues that are expressed, including affective, cognitive, developmental and narrative components (Chazan, 2002). Thus, through play actions, children are able to show and tell their thoughts and feelings when words alone may be insufficient. While play may facilitate conscious thoughts and feelings, it also provides an entry point into unconscious material. *Access to the unconscious* enables the child (or older person) to use defence mechanisms such as projection, displacement, symbolism and/or fantasy to pretend as a process to communicate meaning (Schaefer, 2020). Spontaneous play is informed by implicit memories which may not need to be brought to consciousness. Play provides the medium to externalise internal problems that can be concretely and symbolically expressed. Play also provides opportunities for both *direct teaching*, such as learning to play in new ways to learning a new coping strategy for anxiety, and *indirect teaching*, such as writing a therapeutic story to reframe life events. It was interesting to note that, in the ITEA study within the category 'facilitates communication', specifically *self-expression* was identified to be the most frequently recorded therapeutic power in the puppet play therapy study (Parson, 2017). Alyssa Swan and Sue Bratton (chapter 9) extend on this summary to provide deeper insights into how the TPoP facilitate communication.

Fosters emotional wellness

Catharsis is a psychotherapeutic term used to describe the release of strong emotions including anxiety, stress, anger or fear. In play therapy children may experience play as cathartic when they engage in some physical activities such as hitting or popping a balloon, which allows for the release of muscle tension and negative affect (Schaefer, 2020). *Abreaction* is the term used to describe the reliving of a previous frightening or traumatic experience. It is important for the play therapist to be aware of abreactive play so that the child may be supported to re-create, re-direct and re-experience events through play (Parson & Renshaw, 2017) and in the safety of a therapeutic relationship. Children spontaneously engage in literal or symbolic abreactive play in child-led sessions to foster emotional health and well-being.

Play is fun! Being in a state of play evokes *positive emotions*: feelings of joy, a facial expression with a smile and the sound of laughter are visible cues. Play can be useful for *counterconditioning fears* by gradually exposing an identified fear using specific techniques to desensitise individuals to re-place negative thoughts and feelings with more positive ones. The ther-apeutic powers of play may be activated during *stress inoculation* whereby the play therapist introduces or prepares a child or older person for a po-tentially stressful experience prior to actual real-life experience. An example of this is role-playing going to school for the first time or preparing for a medical procedure. The final TPoP in this section refers to *stress manage-ment* whereby specific play techniques or games can be used to reduce both physical and emotional signs of stress and in some cases distress. Examples of stress management could include creating and colouring in mandalas or zentangles, using fidget or sensory toys and play materials, listening to or playing music and using guided imagery, such as those found via smiling minds app, to help the child relax. Lorri Yasenik (Chapter 10) extends on this summary to provide greater clinical insights into how the TPoP foster emotional wellness.

Enhances social relationship

One of the most significant aspects of play therapy is the development and maintenance of the *therapeutic relationship*. The therapist creates safe, playful and healthy conditions for change by taking a humanistic stance. Carl Rogers (1957, 2012), in his person/client-centred therapy, identified the three core optimal conditions: congruence, unconditional positive regard and empathy. Play therapists are informed by, and embody, these qualities to focus on the child's internal thoughts, feelings and expressions and respond with a genuine, warm and caring attitude. Play facilitates the therapeutic relationship. *Attachment* is the bonding process that initially occurs in the infant–primary caregiver relationship and is experienced within all close re-lationships thereafter. There are four main styles of attachment: secure, in-secure avoidant, insecure ambivalent and disorganised (Ainsworth, Blehar, Waters, & Wall, 1979; Main & Solomon, 1986). In secure and playful in-teractions the therapist delights in the child and demonstrates non-threatening behaviours such as smiling and laughing. These actions replicate early life secure attachment behaviours and aim to enhance and strengthen therapeutic attachment. Attachment behaviours are learnt strategies that provide play therapists with clues to understand the psychosocial needs, wants and wishes of the child. Through pretend role play and specialised peer group play *social competence* can be experienced and explored in order to master social skills and relational interactions. One of the important components of social competence is the ability to understand another's perspective. In play and through sensitive understanding and empathic reflections of the child's thoughts, feelings and concerns the therapist can communicate and role model *empathy*. Ken Gardner (Chapter 11) extends on this summary to provide greater insights into how the TPoP enhance social relationships.

Increases personal strengths

Children never cease to amaze, and, when able to fully immerse and self-initiate play, they will come up with unique and wonderful solutions to problems. Play activates the imagination and facilitates *creative problem solving*. For example, when a toy giraffe family needs to be transported across to the other side of the room or planet and there is no toy truck or plane in sight, the child may use object substitution and a wooden block or a shoe-box could substitute to get the job done. In play, a wide range of unique ideas and stories can be brought to life; these in turn stimulate and extend the imagination to consider alternative possibilities in a safe and carefree way. Another therapeutic effect of play is the development of *resiliency*. Learning to recover from unexpected or difficult situations is a very useful life skill. Some children, and their families, may have to cope with experiences such as parental separation, illness or death of a pet or loved one. When living in a country where frequent natural disasters are common, for example due to floods and fires, building resiliency to cope with such experiences is important. Playing games which involve uncertainty may help in developing resiliency in the early years, games such as snap; rock, paper, scissors or snakes and ladders may sow the seeds for adaptability, flexibility and therefore resiliency. *Moral development* and social conscious may be explored in play. Working out right from wrong, or things being fair or unfair, may be played out in role play where power and control themes or games with rules predominate. Puppets are great fun because the child may freely project onto the puppet and switch positions between being bad or good, kind or mean, rude or smart, but in a safe way that allows the child to show parts of the self and not show the self at the same time.

Vygotsky (1978) stated that 'play creates a zone of proximal development of the child. In play a child always behaves beyond his average age, above his daily behaviour; in play it is as though he were a head taller than himself' (p. 102). This means that children *accelerate psychological development* through play because they are able to extend their play and consider and explore more complex play possibilities without fear. Play can also help foster the mastery of physical, cognitive and emotional regulation. *Self-regulation* is the ability to control impulses and to motivate one-self when bored and calm one-self when hyperaroused. *Self-esteem* is a way of thinking, feeling and acting based on accepting, respecting and believing in own-self (Schaefer, 2020). Through play children can discover their whole self as equal to others. Henry Kronengold (chapter 12) extends on this summary to provide greater insights into how the therapeutic powers of play increases personal strengths.

Conclusion

Play can restore hope, relieve stress, develop problem-solving abilities, allow for a release of emotions and assist in children developing their ability to emotionally regulate. The therapeutic powers of play are a taxonomy of the actual mechanisms which may facilitate or enhance positive change and are used to inform clinical reasoning for specific referrals. I sincerely hope you enjoy the rich insights presented throughout this book, across the landscape, over the EPR continents and to the far-flung reaches of the four corners of the TPoP world.

References

Ainsworth, M. D. S., Blehar, M. C., Waters, E., & Wall, S. (1979). *Patterns of attachment: A psychological study of the strange situation.* ProQuest Ebook Central. Retrieved from https://ebookcentral.proquest.com.

Brown, S. L. (2010). *Play: How it shapes the brain, opens the imagination, and invigorates the soul.* New York, NY: Penguin Group.

Chazan, S. E. (2002). *Profiles of play: Assessing and observing structure and process in play therapy.* London. Jessica Kingsley Publishers.

Drewes, A. A., & Schaefer, C. E. (2014). Introduction: How play therapy causes therapeutic change. In C. E. Schaefer & A. A. Drewes (Eds.), *The therapeutic powers of play: 20 core agents of change.* (2nd ed.). Hoboken, NJ: Wiley.

Eberle, S. G. (2014). The elements of play toward a philosophy and a definition of play. *American Journal of Play, 6,* 214–233.

Hitch, D., Pepin, G. & Stagnitti, K. (2014). The integrating theory, evidence and action (ITEA) method: A procedure for helping practitioners translate theory and research into action. *The British Journal of Occupational Therapy, 77*(12), 592+. doi:10.4276/030802214X14176260335183.

Jennings, S. (1999). *Introduction to developmental playtherapy: Playing and healing.* London: Jessica Kingsley Publishers.

Main, M., & Solomon, J. (1986). Discovery of a new, insecure-disorganized/disoriented attachment pattern. In M. Yogman & T. B. Brazelton (Eds.), *Affective development in infancy* (pp. 95–124). Norwood, NJ: Ablex. [Google Scholar].

Meyer, J. H. F., & Land, R. (2003). Threshold concepts and troublesome knowledge 1 – Linkages to ways of thinking and practising. In C. Rust (Ed.), *Improving student learning – Ten years on.* Oxford: OCSLD.

Parson, J. (2017). *Puppet Play Therapy: Integrating Theory, Evidence and Action.* Presented at the International Play Therapy Study Group Champneys, Forest Mere UK. June 18.

Parson, J., & Renshaw, K. (2017). The therapeutic powers of play. In C. E. Schaefer & A. A. Drewes (Eds.), *The therapeutic powers of play: 20 core agents of change* (2nd ed.). Hoboken, NJ: Wiley. Retrieved from https://www.youtube.com/watch?v=wuu59E97igU.

Rogers, C. (1957). The necessary and sufficient conditions of therapeutic personality change. *Journal of Consulting Psychology, 21*(2), 95–103. Retrieved from https://doi.org/10.1037/h0045357.

Rogers, C. (2012). On person-centered therapy [Video file]. Retrieved August 22, 2019, from https://www.kanopy.com/category/supplier/psychotherapynet.

Schaefer, C. E. (1993). *The therapeutic powers of play*. Northvale NJ: Jason Aronson.

Schaefer, C. E. (2020). *The therapeutic powers of play online training*. Play Therapy Training Institute (PTTI). Retrieved from https://the-play-therapy-training-institute.teachable.com/courses/.

Schaefer, C. E., & Drewes, A. A. (2014). *The therapeutic powers of play: 20 core agents of change* (2nd ed.). Hoboken: John Wiley & Sons, Inc.

Vygotsky, L. S. (1978). *Mind in society: The development of higher psychological processes*. Cambridge, MA: Harvard University Press.

Chapter 2

The EPR informed psychotherapist

Eileen Prendiville

Addressing early wounds in psychotherapy needs more than words: Sue Jennings' (1999) EPR model offers a comprehensive framework to understand the client's presentation, inform our decision making and allow us to practise psychotherapy creatively. This chapter will propose developments of the EPR model and a new framework for the EPR-informed psychotherapist to understand each stage (and additional proposed sub-stages) more fully. This chapter will further understanding of normative development in regard to physical, emotional and role identity; consequences of traumatic stress on children; play associated with each category; associated therapeutic interventions and benefits and how we can use this knowledge to understand and influence the individual psychotherapy process with children and adolescents when play therapy is the medium utilised, and particularly when the child leads the therapy process. Other chapters will provide case examples of children's journeys through the EPR stages.

Introduction

Babies are born into a world full of sensory input and somatic experiencing. Everything is felt more intensely than when inside the womb. There are things to see, hear, taste, touch and smell. More than that, there are sensations arising from within the body. The baby experiences a state of equilibrium when all needs are met, and moves towards distress when a new need arises. The need may be for food, sleep, comfort, adjustments in temperature, relief from pain or simply for help with state regulation. The newborn does not recognise that there is space between self and other. They have no capacity to comfortably delay gratification. They are not logical thinkers – their higher brain regions are not in the driver's seat. Their lower, more primitive, brain regions govern their way of being.

But wait – this infant is already able to agree and disagree! They may move towards what they want and retreat from what they don't want – in effect saying yes and no. They may root to find the breast, accept or reject milk offered by leaning in or pulling back. We want to sustain this capacity. Ideally, this newborn is held, physically and emotionally, by a carer who is responsive to their needs and immature communications and delights in them. The child's early experiences of receiving care implicitly shapes their internal working model of relationships (i.e. attachment style) and informs how they organise knowledge about routine events and sequences as they experience them. These internal scripts shape the child's perceptions of the world and of self. The world view develops based on adaptation to the environment as it is experienced rather than on how these experiences are thought about: it is built on implicit rather than explicit memories.

Responsive and reliable care builds organised sensory systems and a capacity to trust. This is a physical phenomenon – the development of trust is influenced by levels of predictability of receipt of appropriate care and alleviation of distress. Past experience informs expectations for the future. The infant who is reliably restored to a state of balance rather than left in distress learns that distress is temporary, that the world is good, that it is ok to express need and that care is reliably available. This is the basis of trust, and hope is the associated virtue (Erikson, 1968). Trust is at the core of positive mental health and is developed through embodied experiences.

Children with poorly organised sensory systems are prone to sensory misperceptions resulting in inadequate body awareness and integration of self, body and environment (Gaskill & Perry, 2012).

Embodiment-Projection-Role and personal identity

Jennings (1999) describes EPR as a developmental paradigm that uniquely charts the progression of dramatic play, and the dramatised self, from birth to seven years. Despite this short span of years, the paradigm is applicable to individuals throughout the life span and has particular relevance for those in the initial developmental stage and for those who faced challenges at any point in these first seven years. The child progresses through these stages sequentially, each being significantly influenced by the previous stage, any associated disruptions and the degree of maturity achieved. However, all stages remain active so that when a child begins to engage in role play they still engage in both projective and embodiment play. As adults we also engage in embodiment, projective and role activities.

I propose that each of the three identified play areas is directly linked to an important stage in the developmental of personal identity (Prendiville, 2010; Prendiville & Howard, 2017, pp. 22–23).

- physical identity – embodiment play – understanding 'me' as a separate person.
- emotional identity – projective play – understanding personal thoughts, feelings and intentions and becoming aware of 'other'.

- role identity – dramatic and role play – learning to have relationships and develop empathy by developing the ability to see the world from another persons' viewpoint.

Embodiment play is characterised by physical movement and sensory exploration and refinement. Projective play is characterised by the creation of something outside the body: the player imbues meaning onto something external; the internal world is projected out. It includes small world play, story making and artistic creations. Like projective play, role play includes pretend play, but it involves the player in stepping into and developing a role through drama or improvisation.

I have watched Sue work and teach for many years and there is only one conclusion that I can reach about her: she is a creative genius! She has an incredible, exceptional, natural skill and ability in the area of groupwork with people of all ages. She lives and breathes EPR, and her natural habitat is as a leader of a creative group (Jennings, 2014). The location and setting could be anywhere on the planet and any person may be a participant. Sue's sessions are inclusive, there is no set schedule, she adjusts and adapts constantly as she responds to the emerging needs of the group and the individuals within it. The one thing that is constant is her adherence to sequencing – first comes embodiment, then projection and then role play. This is as natural as breathing to Sue. What changes is the theme and the activities as they are responsive to the age and stage of development of the participants and the purpose of the session and/or programme.

Sue's groups may be developmental, educational or therapeutic – at times they are all three. When they include referred clients, they are clearly therapy. One thing is for sure, participants grow and develop through their engagement in the group process, and Sue facilitates this in what appears to be an effortless manner.

Typically, in progressing through the EPR stages, the child become more competent in physical play, small world symbolic play and dramatic play. This equips them in becoming more creative, imaginative and equipped to live fully, joyfully and with greater resilience. Personal development is directly linked to play development.

Should a child experience neglect or trauma, their development may be interrupted and distorted as the usual achievements associated with one or more stages are compromised. This will be influenced both by the stages of development already achieved, the degree to which each has been successfully integrated and by the nature of the trauma, i.e. if it directly confuses or harms the child on a physical, emotional and/or inappropriate role level. Adults who experience trauma will also be affected on these three levels and this will be likewise affected by their earlier experiences at each level so that adult trauma may harm something already achieved (e.g. reduce the ability to trust rather than prevent the ability to trust from developing).

Repeated trauma in adult life erodes the structure of the personality already formed, but repeated trauma in childhood forms and deforms the personality. The child trapped in an abusive environment is faced with formidable tasks of adaptation. She must find a way to preserve a sense of trust in people who are untrustworthy, safety in a situation that is terrifyingly unpredictable, power in a situation of helplessness. Unable to care for or protect herself, she must compensate for the failures of adult care and protection with the only means at her disposal, an immature system of psychological defences.

Dr. Judith Lewis Herman (2015, p. 96)

In contrast to Jennings, the author's natural habitat is individual psychotherapy rather than groupwork. I utilise Sue's EPR model but look through a different lens in attempting to understand what the player's self-directed play is communicating about their struggles. I consider how I can use this to inform clinical decision making and make the most beneficial therapeutic use of myself in the relationship. I suggest that we can use knowledge of early trauma and its impact on personal identity to do the following:

• understand the significance of the child's spontaneous play in therapy.
• understand the self-directed play therapy process (including progress) with children.
• make therapeutic use of self when the therapy process is 'stuck', we see repetitive play without resolution and/or the client needs assistance to progress.

My basic premise is that traumatic, stressful and/or confusing life events interfere with the child's progression through the EPR stages and development of personal identity and may result in the development of behavioral, emotional, and social difficulties. As children best express themselves through play, the child psychotherapist should rely more on understanding what their play is communicating rather than focussing on words. The child's use of verbal language can only inadequately express their experiences and internal processes. It is through play that they share their stories more fully.

The player's engagement in, and possible preoccupation with, embodiment, projective or role play within their play therapy sessions has the potential to inform the therapist's understanding of the area/s of personal identity with which they struggle, the area that distresses them most, the challenges they are attempting to resolve and the stage at which their development was disrupted. Likewise, engagement with parents or carers facilitates the sharing of relevant information about the child's past and their current circumstances.

I have developed Jennings' (1999) model to incorporate a breakdown of her Embodiment stage into three sub-sections, and I explore how interruptions at each of these, plus during the projection and role stages, manifests in difficulties in the child's life, relationships and play capacity. This development of the model further explores how an EPR-based conceptualisation can facilitate understanding play and assist the therapist in making clinical decisions about the player's difficulties and ways to address their needs through play.

The Embodiment stage

Embodiment is the earliest of the stages in the EPR paradigm. The newborn infant does not experience themselves as having a body that is defined and separate from the environment. Children experience the world somatically, via their senses (Norton & Norton, 2006, 2008), and initially express themselves through movement and sound. Their body is their primary means of learning (Jennings, 1999, p. 51), and it is through their physical experiences that they become aware of self, and personal identity begins to develop. The first level is physical identity. The newborn infant has no capacity to meet their own needs: they are totally dependent on others and only very gradually learns to distinguish and process sensory information and gain some degree of control over their own movements. The first stage is involved with the challenges of regulating physiology (with the help of another), learning to recognise and tolerate physical sensations, developing an embodied world view in regard to safety and the reliability of having needs met, capacity to delay gratification, understanding the self as a separate being with personal boundaries and learning if their world is a trustworthy place. How the infant navigates this stage, and the learning that accrues, is closely linked to how reliably needs are met and stress is regulated.

A cycle of need is opened when a child moves from a state of equilibrium towards distress when a need arises. If this need is met quickly, distress is alleviated without causing the child to become overwhelmed and they return to a state of equilibrium. When cycles of need are regularly closed in this way, and the child comes to predict that this is the natural order, they develop trust and a world view based on reliable nurturance and care. Body cues can be noticed, expressed and responded to, setting a firm foundation for the next stage of development. The infant begins to separate out from the primary caregiver in a way that allows them to develop and acknowledge their own boundaries. They begin to develop a bodily sense of 'me and not me', and a sense of 'other'. Successfully negotiating this stage leaves the infant well equipped to respond to both their internal body cues and sensory information outside themselves in a way that facilitates congruence.

Physically intrusive elements of trauma and neglect interfere with physical development and can contribute to sensory dysfunction, lack of awareness of body cues, a lack of co-ordination, and difficulties with personal boundaries. Critically, early and/or significant physical trauma (including neglect) causes:

- difficulties with trust.
- difficulties with saying yes and no.
- personal boundary issues.
- poor body image and low self esteem.

The impacted child will need opportunities to re-connect with their physical self and regain/discover their physical identity in order to develop appropriate feelings of trust and security in the world. Free play sessions, physical and rough and tumble play, embodiment play, developmental movement, nurturing experiences and sensory programmes can provide opportunities for this to happen. Individual needs will be linked to the specific experiences of the child and the earliest E sub-stage (see next paragraph) at which disruptions occurred. Reparative experiences do not have to be therapist directed – the child will bring these into therapy spontaneously when afforded an opportunity to do so. Our job as therapist is to provide an appropriate therapeutic environment, recognise what their play communicates and respond appropriately.

The three proposed sub-stages within the Embodiment stage are these:

1 I am.
2 I can.
3 I am me / I am not you.

Each is involved with achieving increasing levels of understanding 'me' as a separate person.

I am

The first phase, 'I am', is play with motion and the full body. All 'play' with tiny infants takes place within relationship and initially involves the baby's full body. This is what we typically see in nurturing relationships between carer and infant. We bring the infant directly into our space or we move gently, but still intrusively, into theirs. The infant is swaddled, arms and legs are contained within blankets and/or the arms of the carer. We tend to hold infants in a way that provides security – we support their full body and their head – and we use exaggerated safety cues to entice social engagement. We rock them, we pat them, we use patterned movement to soothe. We move our faces close to theirs. We use lilting speech; repetitive, rhythmical sounds; friendly facial expressions and tend to mirror their movements and sounds as if they were a deliberate effort at shared communication. We transmit exaggerated safety cues and draw them into social engagement with us (Kestly, 2014).

In play therapy we watch for children who spontaneously choose 'nesting activities' (e.g. curling in small spaces, getting wrapped in blankets, sandwiching between bean bags), exploratory and sensory play, play with motion, sculpting, nurturing and rough and tumble play to inform us that they need reparative play within this sub-stage.

We can introduce and expand on physical embodiment activities (Sherborne, 2001) to rebalance any developmental (and attachment) issues arising from the 'I am' stage:

- play to foster trust includes all play with motion involving the full body: swinging the child in a blanket or beanbag, rough and tumble play, games of balance, tossing child in air (and catching!), cradling activities where the adult makes a container (between knees, curled in lap) for the child and rocking them, rolling games and sliding games.
- early play that fosters co-operation includes play where the adult and child work together while using full body movement. It includes rocking together, rowing the boat games, balancing with a partner (e.g. pushing to standing or sitting when back to back) and see-saw games.
- play that fosters independence (and assertiveness) includes play where the participants work against each other. Examples are back to back games, 'prison' games where child is captured in the adult's arms and pushes to escape or games where the child is 'a rock' and the adult tries to move them. In 'against' games the adult and child may also swap roles so that the child tries to move the adult. The adult meets the child's strength, encourages effort and allows the child to experience success after they have expended energy.

I can

The second sub-stage in Embodiment is known as 'I can' and involves demonstration of all that the child can now do with their body. It includes gaining head control and mastering movement from the midline such as pulling the self to a sitting position and rolling from back to front and vice versa. This phase builds on foundations laid in the 'I am' phase and corresponds with the stage when infants are learning to control their bodies, regulate their breathing, and make deliberate movements including intentionally moving arms and legs, picking up and releasing objects, passing objects from hand to hand and developing gross and fine motor skills. The child has grown from simple awareness of *being* into a more complex awareness of *doing*. When children learn, experientially, about what they can physically do, there sense of identity and autonomy grows. This facilitates self-esteem and self-confidence. Interruptions in this stage negatively impact on self-concept as part of the developing world view. A child may be exposed to too much or too little risk in terms of being free to explore safely and return to a safe base

(Jennings, 1999, pp. 91–98). Fear may impede exploration, or unfortunate circumstances, such as injury, illness or an impoverished environment, may prevent the child being afforded opportunities to develop physical skills and associated self-confidence. Developmental trauma during this period is particularly disruptive.

When provided with an accepting play therapy experience within a facilitating environment, children struggling with lowered self-efficacy in regard to their physical identity often spontaneously choose to play 'circus' games and sporting activities, and they demonstrate their physical skills and strength. We see lots of movement: ball play, boxing, tumbling, crawling, climbing, balancing and negotiating obstacle courses. We may also see breathwork activities – blowing bubbles and balloons. Controlled breathwork lays firm foundations for the later regulation of emotion in the P stage.

Therapeutic activities in the *I can* sub-stage focus on using the body parts and on increasing awareness of how the body works and moves. There will be a focus on movement. Lots of embodiment activities, including movement games involving the weight-bearing and the non-weight-bearing parts of the body, are detailed in Veronica Sherborne's *Developmental Movement for Children* book. They include funny walks, disappearing knee tricks, walking on knees, walking when squatting down, high knee walking and lots more (Sherborne, 2001).

Individual play may also include baby games that heighten awareness of body parts, for example counting fingers and toes, safe massage, pushing and pulling, games like clap hands, round and round the garden and tickling. These games also build a capacity to tolerate excitement/anxiety, anticipation and support self-regulation.

I am me/ I am not you

The final sub-stage in Embodiment is known as 'I am me/I am not you'. This is the stage at which the child explores boundaries and learns, experientially, that they are a totally separate physical being. The essence of this stage is experiencing the skin as a boundary, a container for self, through engagement with materials of varying textures, temperatures and degrees of messiness. This stage is a bridge into projective play as it involves materials outside the body. However, the materials are explored in the context of experiencing sensations on the skin, learning 'where I end' rather than as elements in a constructed story. This lays the groundwork for tolerating and respecting personal space, developing autonomy, individuality and avoiding enmeshment with others. It builds the child's capacity to be separate, self-contained and authentic.

Difficulties in this sub-stage lead to confusion about the need for personal space and how this is linked to degrees of intimacy. Those who do not satisfactorily negotiate this stage do not fully experience themselves as separate beings. There may be ongoing confusion in regard to recognising and reading physiological sensations – difficulties in adequately recognising or responding to body cues that are linked to hunger or satiation, heat or cold or to the sensations in their body that are linked to recognising emotions and developing emotional intelligence. The individual may find themselves more equipped to attune to the emotions of others than to their own internal life and find themselves ill-prepared to recognise, acknowledge and value their own thoughts and feelings within the P stage. There are also long-term impacts on the subsequent R stage as those who struggle in this area are prone to invade others' space inappropriately, may experience the response as rejecting and develop traits that are perceived as defiant. Alternatively, there may be a risk of proneness to enmeshed relationships.

Activities in the 'I am me, I am not you' sub-phase focus on experiencing the skin as a boundary and with learning to recognise the textural and other properties of objects through contact with the skin. Therefore it is involved with lots of sensory, tactile sensations and messy play. Play with sand, water, mud, gloop, wet clay, and use of finger (and foot, elbow, knee!) painting is useful. Play with textures and temperature is important. The aim is that the child develops an increased awareness of its boundaries. Embodiment play with substances are not designed to create an aesthetically pleasing product – the materials are engaged with purely from a sensory point of view (Prendiville & Fearn, 2017).

Benefits of embodiment play in child psychotherapy

Reparative embodiment play is important to counteract physical identity issues; to foster development of a healthy physical sense of self, positive self-image and self-efficacy; to support the development of trust and secure attachment; to develop appropriate boundaries and to lay foundations for emotional development and engagement in healthy relationships.

It develops the ability to read body cues, recognise physiological needs, achieve better co-ordination and reduce physical rigidity and body armouring. It facilitates taking an assertive stance and makes 'no' possible. Practicing working with and working against others develops the capacity to be resistant, prevents co-dependency and inappropriate confluence and facilitates groundedness, physiological regulation, calmness and containment. The capacity to trust our intuition and be creative and spontaneous has its roots in the Embodiment stage. This is at the core of a neurosequential approach to neurobiologically informed creative psychotherapy (Prendiville & Howard, 2017).

The Projective stage

Projective play typically predominates for children aged one to three years and continues throughout childhood and beyond. It is characterised by the use of materials outside the body and the child's emerging ability for pretence, narrative and sequencing. It is important for developing emotional identity and emotional boundaries, establishing a sense of security in the world and enhancing the ability to make sense of experiences. Children need to actively explore and learn experientially rather than by rote techniques: they need to manipulate three-dimensional objects to learn about the world and to develop concepts – especially children under seven years who are still in Piaget's pre-operational stage (Piaget, 1962). Projective play enriches the child's emotional vocabulary and promotes the development of emotional intelligence which has been found to be more important to a child than IQ, and it is a better indicator of future success (Goleman, 1996).

Pretend play opens a window into the child's inner world: 'The child is projecting ideas and feelings into the toys and objects' (Jennings, 1999, p. 101); play with small world toys gives the player 'an opportunity to exercise control over their world rather than being overwhelmed with epic size experiences' (p. 6). It is in this stage of dramatic development that the child begins to learn more about the world outside themselves, to manipulate objects, to see what things can do (and have done to them!). They develop imaginative, verbal and cognitive skills. In addition to small world play, projective play includes play with objects (e.g. construction play), art and craft activities, story-making, and any creative expression where the child produces a picture or symbol. Creations tell us something about the personality, world view and current preoccupations of the creator. This brings it into the emotional domain. Basically, this type of play involves the player in taking something from their inner world, externalising it to make it visible and separate from themselves and perhaps doing something with it now that it can be more easily actively explored and understood. When children engage in such play, they make sense of their experiences, learning about their own emotions and the world around them, and gain understanding of their own, and others', thoughts, feelings, intentions and actions. Whatever is confusing for the child will find its way into the stories they create.

Just as the projective stage follows on from embodiment, the development of emotional identity has its roots in physical identity. Children's beginning interest in projective play, late in the first year of life, accompanies their growing capacity to use their body intentionally and growing awareness of physiological cues. Emotional development is concerned with recognising emotions and learning to express these congruently and appropriately. A key foundation is awareness of the sensations in our bodies: emotions arise from within; feelings have a physical component. Learning to understand these physical cues in terms of their emotions is core to P, the second stage in the EPR paradigm.

Unpredictable elements of developmental trauma interfere with emotional development, distort the child's emotional sense of self and cause the following:

- difficulties with making sense of physiological sensations and understanding emotions.
- hyper-arousal, overwhelming emotions and perhaps hypo-arousal.
- confusion.
- difficulties with sequencing.
- difficulties with memory, including intrusive recollections.

The child needs opportunities to develop an emotional vocabulary, become emotionally literate and get in touch with their true needs and feelings. Projective play with stories, sand, art, small world toys and puppets can provide opportunities for this to happen. Children need opportunities to make stories and play sequences with clear stages of beginning, middle and end. The as-if qualities of symbolic play are particularly important in facilitating the child's healing and development.

Benefits of projective play in child psychotherapy

Projective play in therapy provides opportunities for the child to project their own stories, hopes, dreams, fears, and confusions onto material outside their body where it can be engaged with externally. Repetitive play themes, the degree of order or disorder evident and the presence or absence of shifts and resolution informs the therapist about therapeutic progress.

Sand play therapy, creating situations with miniature objects, art activities and play with puppets lend themselves to facilitating projective play. When a child creates a story, they learn about sequencing, about beginnings, middles and endings. This provides emotional containment for the content of the story. Physical containment, and additional safety, can also be provided by the use of a sandtray or page, a tent or other enclosed space. The therapeutic relationship and use of play make it possible for unresolved material to be safely explored. It is in creating stories that children project out their fears, anxieties, confusions and current concerns. They are most likely to do this symbolically, using metaphors to provide emotional distance. This happens on an unconscious level and is useful in providing the dramatic distance that paradoxically allows the creator of the story to get closer to what is preoccupying them at the time. Making the story brings the child closer to understanding the thoughts, feelings and intentions of others and also allows the child to learn more about their own emotions and how they might differ from those of others. Exploring inner material that has been externalised allows the creator to learn more about it, to become less confused and less preoccupied with it and to make sense of the emotions attached to it.

Dramatic distance and the associated 'as if' quality allows even traumatic memories to be more fully engaged with, emotional intensity is reduced and change becomes possible. The emotional tone connected to memories can be transformed, new endings envisaged, confusion replaced with clarity, disorganisation is replaced with sequencing and experiences of disempowerment and being overwhelmed can be emotionally digested.

The Role stage

Children begin to engage in simple role play in their third year. Role play can be described as dramatised projective play. This stage differs from the projective stage in that the player enacts and develops the role directly rather than ascribing it to characters in small world play or stories. Play with puppets can be the bridge from the P to the R stage as the child partially inhabits the puppet character by moving their limbs and/or giving them a voice. This facilitates the transition to role play which has its foundations in both the E and P stages with the associated development of physical and emotional identity which pave the way for role identity formation.

By stepping into the role of another in play, the child first embodies the character. They attempt to understand them on a physical level and dramatise this – e.g. hunching over as an old woman, standing tall as a royal figure. They combine this physical identification with an emotional identification – reading body cues to get a sense of what the character might be feeling and how they would act. Then they put this into motion – acting out the role, doing what they think the other would do, learning about the 'why' and the 'how' of what the other does, all the time learning how it feels to be this 'other' on a physical and emotional level. When children engage in socio-dramatic play (role play with others) they can also learn how the other characters are affected by and respond to the character that they are portraying. Such play enables the child to make sense of their world, learn more about the world from another's perspective, to understand relationships, develop communication skills, and increase their ability to engage in meaningful interactions with others. It provides opportunities to communicate with peers, develop negotiation skills, learn to share, take/give the lead, move from onlooker and solitary play to parallel, associative and eventually to co-operative play. The ability to empathise is developed. Gaskill (2014, p. 202) highlights the power of role play in the development of empathy:

> With each reenactment, the child becomes more socially aware, knowledgeable, and adept regarding how each character thinks, feels, and responds in a social context. With further neurological growth, new skills and social competencies become possible (sharing, taking turns, and demonstrating respect), all needing to be honed through dramatic play.

Children often prefer to take the powerful position when engaged in role play. They are trying to learn about being powerful in a world where adults are in charge and socio-dramatic play facilitates this. Less powerful roles (e.g. the baby, the patient) are often assigned to dolls or to children who are trying to establish their place in the group. In other games, the roles switch regularly so that each child gets opportunities to be in all positions according to some recognised structure (e.g. in hide and seek, tag, skipping games).

The content of the scenes children create arise from their day to day life, from material they are attempting to assimilate, and from unresolved issues in their past. Children learn about roles in their interactions and relationships with others and by witnessing relationships in the world they inhabit. The microsystems in which they live have the greatest influence on their development of role identity, and their expectations of traditional roles (e.g. what a mother is, what a father does, how grandparents behave, how children are meant to be, etc.). They learn who they are, what is expected of them and how they are perceived by what they see reflected in the eyes of those who interact with them. This can be positive or negative: a cherished daughter, a troublemaker, a bad student, a nuisance, a child who is loved however they are or one who is only accepted, and therefore acceptable, if behaving in a certain way. Children may adopt a false self to try to secure approval and positive, or any, attention – a clown, a caregiver, a scholar etc. This prevents the child being fully true to themselves and authentic in their relationships.

Children may be deliberately involved in harmful relationships and assigned roles, such as a sexual partner, or given inappropriate responsibilities, such as taking care of an adult's mental health, which are confusing, developmentally inappropriate and harmful to them. Interpersonal trauma, which often includes emotional abuse, significantly interrupts healthy role development and places the child in an intolerable situation in which they are often trapped. Interpersonal trauma may also include physical or sexual abuse, exposure to domestic violence and/or neglect. Each of these will also impact on all levels of personal identity. The degree of impact will be related to the age and stage of development achieved by the child when the trauma occurred, and by the presence or absence of attuned, responsive and available caregivers at the time.

If such trauma occurs in the context of a primary attachment relationship the lens through which the child views themselves, others and the world becomes distorted. Most significantly, if such trauma also impacted on the earlier E and P stages, the child will not have had opportunities to sufficiently develop their physical and emotional identity and the impact on their role identify will be even more severe. Self-image is influenced by the image we see reflected in those we share our lives with.

Inappropriate roles in childhood cause the following:

- difficulties with understanding the thoughts and feelings of others.
- difficulties with developing empathy.
- role confusion and distorted thinking in regard to relationships.
- difficulties with social and emotional development.

Children can benefit from a number of perspectives in role play: playing a role assigned and written by another, playing or interacting with a character in a role that is responding spontaneously to another character, or playing a self-directed, central, character in a drama that is their own production. The greatest healing comes from enacting self-constructed scenes as this provides opportunities to explore personally relevant issues. The themes and content of such play may be informed by implicit memories, be symbolic in form and abreactive in nature (Prendiville, 2014). When a therapist engages in socio-dramatic play with a child and takes all direction from the child, allowing the child to lead and tell the adult what to say and what to do, they allow the child to be the writer, producer and director of the scene and the adult is an actor. In this way the child gets personal benefit from the play as they explore the issues relevant to themselves – rather than the adult's issues! Should this play become repetitive, remaining static and without resolution or repair, the child is indicating that they need additional help to resolve the issue they are attempting to address (Prendiville, 2014). At such times, and in recognition that the child has created the experience for the therapist as part of their play and that the child is likely to have cast the therapist in a role that is familiar, and unresolved, to the child, the therapist may draw on their own internal somatic experience to respond spontaneously to the character played by the child. Such therapeutic use of self is also informed by the therapist's knowledge of the child, the stage in the therapy process and the child's past and current circumstances (Prendiville, 2014, p. 95). Giving language to the immediate sensory and somatic aspects of the assigned role, at the time that the child has, probably unconsciously, provoked these in the therapist, supports integration and resolution, addresses confusion and builds connection between the right and left hemispheres.

Benefits of role play in child psychotherapy

In role play children learn about themselves in relation to others, become aware of the feelings and perspectives of others, gain understanding of their own assigned roles and practice new roles for the future. Role play is essential in developing the capacity for empathy. It brings physical and emotional identity together: it involves the joint activation of embodiment and projective play in exploration of role identity.

As it involves the full body, rather than small toys, and the feelings are dramatised rather than ascribed, it allows the child the greatest opportunities to move away from any inappropriate role they learned and any compromising manner of coping. In non-directive therapy children may spontaneously create scenes and stories and enact themes of confusion, injustice, power/control, being trapped, trickery, fear/terror or rescue. Traumatised children gain empowerment over overwhelming emotions and benefit from the alternative viewpoint afforded by stepping into a different role.

Role play is particularly useful in helping the child to overcome any inappropriate sense of shame, guilt or responsibility and to move from being in the 'victim' role. Dramatic distance within the play allows the child to take risks that lead to increased assertiveness, self-confidence and self-assurance.

EPR in the therapy process

I have found that the EPR paradigm can be invaluable in tracking the therapy process. Children may initially play predominantly in one category giving clues as to the areas in which they experience greatest distress (see Table 2.1). This may be different than the area of concern raised by the referrer. For example, a parent may describe a lack of friends as the presenting problem, but the child's projective play may indicate that they are struggling more with confusion over life events. Or a parent may be most concerned by the child's bullying behaviour, and the child's embodiment play may suggest that they are struggling with managing boundaries.

Exploring the child's background (and learning of their experiences, how they responded to potentially traumatic or confusing events and how responsive their environment was, and is, to their needs, communications and miscommunications) provides further context. Getting a vivid description of the child's concerning behaviours, and the contexts in which these occur, provides further clues as to the nature of the child's struggles and their primary therapeutic needs. I believe that 'problem behaviours' are really the child's best efforts to cope when overwhelmed. Considering at what age this behaviour might be age appropriate (e.g. toddler-style tantrums) gives us further clues into the stage at which their struggles began or intensified. Working in partnership with relevant adults in the child's life enables us to support them in supporting the child in a developmentally appropriate manner that is linked to *stage* rather than *chronological age* and provides valuable information for the therapist also.

If a parent presents a history of early neglect, perhaps linked to institutional care in infancy, we can hypothesise that the child will have struggles with some or all three embodiment sub-stages. However, the child may be most upset by a lack of friends and so their play may start in the R category. This does not mean that they have successfully negotiated the E and P stages, it simply indicates that the current area of distress for the child is in

Table 2.1 Summary of EPR sequence with personal identity and potential struggles

Category	Area of personal identity	Struggle
Embodiment	Physical	Boundaries
Projective	Emotional	Confusion
Role	Role	Relationships

their struggles with relationships. Early play in therapy indicates the struggle. Healing begins when we see the child move back through the stages. This may be sequential, moving through *projective* play, then *I am me/I am not you* play, to *I can* play and finally *I am* play, or they may jump straight back to one of the E sub-stages. The child will move back to the earliest stage when development was disrupted, or where their needs were so poorly met that they could not achieve satisfactory embedding of the associated area of personal identity. Reparative play at this level is the key to healing. As each stage builds on foundations laid at the previous stage, therapy will also address each subsequent phase. Noting the progression through these stages enables the therapist to track the therapy process and make clinical decisions as appropriate if the process becomes stuck or the child needs the environment adjusted to afford opportunities for the various phases. To this end, the EPR-informed psychotherapist ensures that the playroom is equipped appropriately to allow for reparative embodiment, projective and role play.

As the child heals there will be fewer play disruptions, more coherence, a lessening of intensity, more resolution in stories, less negative emotions, less repetition and a greater sense of spontaneity apparent in the play session. The child is likely to have renegotiated all three stages in the EPR paradigm: embodiment-projection-role.

References

Erikson, E. (1968). *Identity: youth and crisis*. New York: W.W. Norton & Company.

Gaskill, R., & Perry, B. D. (2012). Child sexual abuse, traumatic experiences, and their impact on the developing brain. In P. Goodyear-Brown (Ed.), *Child sexual abuse: Identification, assessment, and treatment* (pp. 29–47). Hoboken, NJ: Wiley.

Gaskill, R. (2014). Empathy. In A. A. Drewes & C. E. Schaefer (Eds.), *The therapeutic powers of play* (2nd ed., pp. 195–209). New Jersey: Wiley.

Goleman, D. (1996). *Emotional intelligence: Why it can matter more than IQ*. UK: Bloomsbury Publishing PLC.

Herman, J. (2015). *Trauma and recovery*. New York: Basic Books.

Jennings, S. (1999). *An introduction to developmental playtherapy*. London: Jessica Kingsley.

Jennings, S. (2011). *Healthy attachments and neuro-dramatic-play*. London: Jessica Kingsley.

Jennings, S. (2014). Applying an embodiment-projection-role framework in groupwork with children. In E. Prendiville & J. Howard (Eds.), *Play therapy today: Contemporary practice for individuals, groups, and parents* (pp. 81–96). London, England: Routledge.

Kestly, T. A. (2014). *The interpersonal neurobiology of play: Brain-building interventions for emotional well-being*. New York: Norton & Co.

Norton, C., & Norton, B. E. (2006). Experiential play therapy. In C. E. Schaefer & H. G. Kaduson (Eds.), *Contemporary play therapy: Theory, research, and practice* (pp. 28–54). New York, NY: Guilford Press.

Norton, C., & Norton, B. E. (2008). *Reaching children through play therapy: An experiential approach* (3rd ed.). Denver: White Apple Press.

Piaget, J. (1962). *Play, dreams, and imitation in childhood*. London: Routledge.

Prendiville, E. (2010). The play therapy process: Interventions with children with attachment difficulties. Key note address. *Romanian Play Therapy and Dramatherapy Association Annual International Conference, Brasov, 2 October 2010*.

Prendiville, E. (2014). Abreaction. In C. E. Schaefer & A. A. Drewes (Eds.), *The therapeutic powers of play: 20 core agents of change* (2nd edn, pp. 83–102). New Jersey: Wiley & Sons.

Prendiville, E., & Howard, J. (2017). Neurobiologically informed psychotherapy. In E. Prendiville & J. Howard (Eds.), *Creative psychotherapy: Applying the principles of neurobiology to play and expressive arts-based practice* (pp. 21–38). Oxen: Routledge.

Prendiville, S., & Fearn, M. (2017). Coming alive: Finding joy through sensory play. In E. Prendiville & J. Howard (Eds.), *Creative psychotherapy: Applying the principles of neurobiology to play and expressive arts-based practice* (pp. 121–137). Oxon: Routledge.

Sherborne, V. (2001). *Developmental movement for children*. London: Worth Publishers.

Chapter 3

Integrating the therapeutic powers of play in clinical practice settings

Paris Goodyear-Brown

Worldwide data points to the increased prevalence in mental health needs for children and adolescents (De la Barra, 2009). More than half of mental health issues begin in childhood or adolescents (Kessler et al., 2005) and continue into adulthood. Children with specific mental health diagnoses have historically been taken to outpatient clinics for individual, group or family therapy services. However, play-based interventions are now being utilised in a variety of settings, including hospitals (Burns-Nader & Hernandez-Reif, 2016), schools (Green & Christensen, 2006; Ray, Armstrong, Balkin, & Jayne, 2015) and homes and by a variety of helping professionals (play therapists, counsellors, social workers, teachers, marriage and family therapists, occupational therapists, child-life specialists and speech pathologists (Couch, Deitz, & Kanny, 1998).

In this chapter, we will discuss both the design of space and the specific therapeutic powers of play that are facilitated by developmentally sensitive clinical play therapy spaces. After 20 years of adapting sterile school, office and clinic environments to the needs of children, I set out to create a home-like, play house environment that would quickly soothe the reptilian brain stem and the limbic brain of children and teens in ways that answered the questions 'am I safe?' and 'am I loved?' with resounding yeses. Nurture House, our child and family treatment centre located in Franklin, Tennessee, is the most current expression of how we harness the therapeutic powers of play in physical space. This home-like environment invites a neuroception of safety more quickly than traditional practice settings. From the colours on the wall to the titrations of bigness and smallness in physical space (Goodyear-Brown, 2019) to the smells, sounds and textures that are tuned to the needs of individual clients. We have diffusers for use in every room of Nurture House and keep a kit of essential oils that allows families to explore the scents that are most upregulating or downregulating for them. We expand, throughout the course of treatment, the client's ability to check in with their own bodies to know whether they need up-or-down regulating and support them in asking for smells, tastes, or other sensory experiences they may need. We keep a giant gumball machine with free gum in the hallway, so that children have access to this tool for providing pro-prioceptive and vestibular input to the lower brain regions so that ther-apeutic movement can be maximised during treatment. Most rooms have some form of snuggle nook, as we do an enormous amount of attachment enhancement work, helping parents and children delight in one another again. Even within these cosy spots, the softness of blankets offered and the variety of fabrics and textures (rough, smooth, slippery, bumpy) are in-tentionally chosen to offer choice and provide the kind of sensory input that a child or teen might need to regulate through challenging play scenarios.

Piaget conceptualised play patterns that allow for active experimentation and the invitation for repetition of behaviours, skills or stories to aid in the mental digestion of new experiences (1969). Charles Schaefer began ar-ticulating the therapeutic powers of play decades ago and others have built on his work since. The therapeutic powers are grouped, roughly, into four main categories: therapeutic powers of play that facilitate communication, those that foster emotional wellness, those that increase personal strengths, and those that enhance social relationships (see Figure 1.1).

All aspects of a child's development are naturally stimulated through play. Therefore, any area of developmental delay or immaturity in a specific developmental arena (cognitive, physical, social emotional, etc) is aided by the incorporation of play into the pursuit of growth. As children do not develop the ability to think abstractly until around puberty, in a fully equipped play-room the toys become their words and the play becomes their conversation (Hall, Kaduson, & Schaefer, 2002). Whether we approach the therapeutic benefits of play through an attachment lens, a neurobiological lens, a social learning lens, a skills enhancement lens, a trauma recovery lens or a resiliency lens, play is critical for healthy development. More specifically, play can aid in growth trajectories related to a myriad of mental health issues.

The standard delivery of play therapy occurs in a single room or two. These rooms can be set apart spaces within a school building, within a hospital, within a private practice setting or within a community mental health centre. In some cases, a therapist is taking a play therapy kit into a family's home, and, in some school-based settings, therapists are using whatever space is available, evidencing extreme flexibility by meeting with children in spaces as small as a utility closet to spaces as large as the school gymnasium. An important dynamic to consider when the therapeutic powers of play are being activated is the bigness or smallness of the space (Goodyear-Brown, 2019). Felt safety is needed for children to begin taking risks that lead to growth. To that end, making sure that our play spaces are communicating safety and the appropriate level of containment for the child in our care is foundational.

Arming ourselves with a rich understanding of bottom-up brain devel-opment also helps us scaffold the therapeutic uses of play based on which areas of development must be targeted first. In many cases, children are referred for therapeutic work due to big behaviours – crying, screaming, tantruming, bouts of aggression, etc. In other cases, children may present with an anxious, constricted affect or physical state. These children may be aided by utilising play to bring them more deeply into their bodies. In both clinical presentations, one early focus of treatment will include expanding the window of tolerance, often through cycles of upregulating and down-regulating. This is where the therapeutic powers of play really shine.

Play allows for a titrated approach to whatever growing edge (Vygotsky, 1987) is needed for a child. The child who needs to connect mind to body more deeply may benefit from an environment that invites jumping, throwing, skipping and other kinds of full body engagement. Other children may need to practise sitting in stillness and may benefit from small, calming spaces with very few toys. In these cases, early work may focus on devel-oping safety and helping to regulate the lower brain regions. Since pro-prioception and the vestibular sense are both experienced and encoded in our lower brain regions, making sure that we are providing experiences that match the child's unique sensory profile sets the stage for other therapeutic powers of play to be harnessed. Interoception, our ability to interpret the cues inside our bodies as we navigate the world around us, becomes an important focal point for our use of space in clinical settings. To this end, Nurture House has been intentional about the choice of toys for each room and intentional around the design of clinical spaces.

Our continual goal is to give children options: both big spaces and small spaces, and very contained spaces within larger spaces so that we can match the therapeutic space chosen for work to optimise the therapeutic powers of play while allowing us to follow the child's need. Some of this need can be assessed even in the lobby or waiting room of the clinical setting. Part of our initial dyadic assessments begins with a careful observation of a child and parent's behaviour in the lobby. Some children are sitting in the tiny little leather chairs and others may be rolling around on the floor or jumping from grown-up chair to grown-up chair. A parent and child may be snuggled together reading a book on a sofa bench large enough for two and other parents and children may have chosen to wait far apart from one another in the lobby. On occasion we even have grown-ups who wiggle themselves down into the tiny, leather, child-sized chairs. This initial presentation can give us valuable information about the needs of the client. The parent who is waiting in children's chairs may be communicating a need for more containment and may experience the neuro-ception of safety most quickly in a room that provides a sense of smallness or snugness. Children who are already engaged in gross motor play in the lobby may be most easily engaged and transitioned by moving immediately to our sensory room, where jumping from sensory squares to a small trampoline and into the ball pit meets the movement needs of the child.

It is important to honour the feelings of fear, awkwardness or self-consciousness that parents and children may bring with them as they are entering clinical settings. Traditionally, clinic settings have followed a medical model of design: large, open lobbies with rows of chairs, tables with adult magazines, and perhaps a television which may be playing sports, news, or other content that may or may not be appropriate for children. Shiny cold floors and fluorescent lights have also traditionally been the norm in mental health spaces. Children and families who are coming for clinical help already feel pathologised. Children may be expecting something punitive or lecturing but when they are greeted with a home-like environment where play is invited, even in the waiting room, they begin to let down their guard. In terms of the therapeutic powers of play, simply having toys in the lobby invites positive emotion and stress inoculation (two of the powers in the category of fostering emotional wellness).

While toys that encourage kinesthetic manipulation may be most appropriate for the lobby, toys that are likely to activate unconscious content or trauma processing are not. Since play is the natural language of children, we want to approach their therapeutic play invitations like we would approach conversations with adults: Some conversations are for public places and some require privacy. Ginott's famous statement (1960), 'Play is their talk and toys are their words' challenges us to make sure that we are selecting toys based on what a child needs to express. Beginning play therapists will often ransack attics and yard sales for toys for their playrooms. While toys found at garage sales and thrift stores can be powerful tools in a child's therapeutic work, toys for therapeutic spaces should be *selected* not *collected* (Landreth, 1993).

The specific toys offered to harness the therapeutic powers of play may vary based on the theoretical orientation or treatment model of the clinician.

Selected toys should be fairly durable, easy to clean, allow for self-expression and offer points of contact with the therapist. A fully equipped therapeutic playroom includes certain standard categories of toys that invite various therapeutic powers of play. Certain kinds of play should be invited – including messy play, sensory play, aggressive play, nurturing play, post-traumatic play, self-regulation play and attachment enhancement play. Broad categories of toys include toys that pull for nurture or engagement in real-life scenarios, toys that allow for the expression of aggression and toys that allow for creative expression. There is a fairly universal set of toys and tools that are needed when outfitting a play therapy space. There are some tweaks and nuances based on which model of play therapy you are using, but there is general agreement around certain categories of tools. Schaefer and Drewes (2013) argue that the therapeutic powers of play are transtheoretical. To this end, a cross-section of toys that will be seen in a therapeutic playroom will be used by the child-centred play therapist (Landreth, 2012), the Adlerian play therapist (Kottman and Meany-Walen, 2015), or the TraumaPlay therapist (Goodyear-Brown, 2010, 2019, 2021) alike. Helping professionals from different theoretical orientations may lean more heavily on certain core agents of change in the use of play; for example, a humanistic clinician may value self-expression as the most important change agent in play therapy, while a psychoanalytic play therapist may see abreaction and catharsis as primary healing mechanisms. Below is a beginning, but certainly not exhaustive, list of the kinds of toys in each of these three categories that will invite the therapeutic powers of play to be activated in clinical settings. Regardless of theoretical orientation or clinical setting, a basic play therapy kit is likely to include many of the items listed in the table below.

The reader will note that, in the category of aggressive toys, the bop bag and pretend guns both appear with a caveat that their inclusion may vary depending on the theoretical orientation of the clinician harnessing the therapeutic powers of play. Some clinicians feel that inviting aggressive expressions, allowing for acting out in the safe presence of the clinician provides therapeutic benefits to the client including catharsis or abreaction (both therapeutic powers of play in the category of fostering emotional wellness). Other clinicians believe that allowing children to engage in re-petitions of aggressive actions, particularly the hitting or kicking of the bop bag, may be deepening the neural pathways towards aggression as a maladaptive expression of big feelings. These clinicians believe that parti-cularly for children who are already given to impulsivity and aggressive expressions, the pleasure of aggressive discharge might further enhance the aggression, not 'cathart' it. Some therapists use an approach that still allows for aggressive expression, i.e. throwing wet cotton balls to stick on the wall while they verbalise something related to their anger. This allows for the kinaesthetic aggression (body) to be paired with the verbal (cognitive) ex-pression, helping to integrate mind and body. This approach may

Table 3.1 Toys that pull for aggression

Creative expression	Nurture/real life/role play	Aggression/post-traumatic play
Crayons/markers/ paper	Baby dolls/baby bottles	Play swords
Sand/water	Puppets (nurturing, aggressive, vulnerable)	Play knives
Clay	Doll house/doll family	Handcuffs
Paints	Dress up clothes	Bop bag (varies based on theoretical orientation)
Art supplies	Doctor's kit	Army men
Magic wands	Kitchen/play food/utensils	Jail
Mirror	Cash register	Length of rope
Building blocks	Play money	Pretend guns (varies depends of theoretical orientation)
Musical instruments	Telephones	Balls

encourage the catharsis of anger as opposed to the recycling or reinforcement of aggressive impulses.

The question about whether or not to have guns in the playroom also sparks some debate. For the child who lives in a violent neighbourhood and has witnessed gun violence, or perhaps sees older kids and adults carrying guns, having a safe space in which to be in charge of the guns may be experienced as empowering. My first playroom, in a therapeutic preschool setting in a community mental health centre, included little orange dart guns. Memorable experiences in which children used the guns to exert power and control over any of the toys in the playroom that seemed dangerous to them by shooting them (and sometimes having me shoot them too) helped to quickly establish enough neuroception of safety in the physical space that they took risks (to speak, to connect, to approach traumatic content) that they had not been able to take before (Goodyear-Brown, 2010). Later, I moved into a public school setting with a strict zero tolerance policy in force that did not allow for weapons of any kind on the premises, pretend or real. What I found quickly is that children will make a gun (with Legos, with the legs of a Barbie or with their fingers) if they need one in their play. Traumatised children, who have experienced helplessness and victimisation at the hands of someone more powerful, will often enter into role plays with the weapons. They will set up play scenarios in which the therapist is asked to play the victim. This can become profound re-enactment and allow children to experience the fulfilment of a fantastical wish for destructive power, and frequently ends in a discarding of the role of perpetrator. Role plays of this kind, and all kinds really, help children take the perspective of another, and in this way can help grow empathy, another therapeutic power of play and social competence while sometimes helping to accelerate their psychological development, another therapeutic power of play.

In this form of play, limit setting becomes very important. Since no one is actually being hurt, therapists are encouraged to remain in role, often verbalising the probable thoughts/feelings that a victim in this situation would have. However, if the child violates a boundary the clinician must be able to come quickly out of role, kindly and calmly set the boundary, and move right back into role. There are times in this kind of aggressive role play when the child takes the role of victim and asks you to play the powerful person, perhaps even the perpetrator. Again, limit setting is critically important in this sort of play, as any request from the child to actually re-enact abusive moments must be met with education about the role of 'safe bosses'. I will often don some sort of silly costume piece when asked to play a perpetrator role, to further distinguish myself as safe boss and play partner from the role in which I have been put. There have been many scenarios in which I have been instructed to 'act mean', put the child in jail or in a locked room and then been instructed to 'fall asleep' while they break out of jail, eat the pretend food they make for me and 'be poisoned and die!' Harnessing the imagination, children who are working through trauma will play through multiple scenarios that ultimately provide them a sense of empowerment and freedom.

Real life and re-enactment play

When children are given a full set of toys that mirror the home environment, including a play kitchen with play dishes, play foods, babies, a baby bottle, a stroller, a high chair, an iron and ironing board, these items invite a child to play out real-life scenarios. Self-expression, a seminal therapeutic power of play, is fostered when these tools are offered. We may be able to tell a lot about the nurture a child has received by observing the ways in which they nurture or take care of the baby dolls (see Figure 3.1).

Abreaction, a therapeutic power of play that is sometimes misunderstood, is a term that is rooted in a psychoanalytic tradition. It is a term for re-living the traumatic experience to leach out the emotional toxicity. Some describe it as a process of desensitisation. In play therapy, the toys provide potentially abreactive opportunities. As the verbal language of children

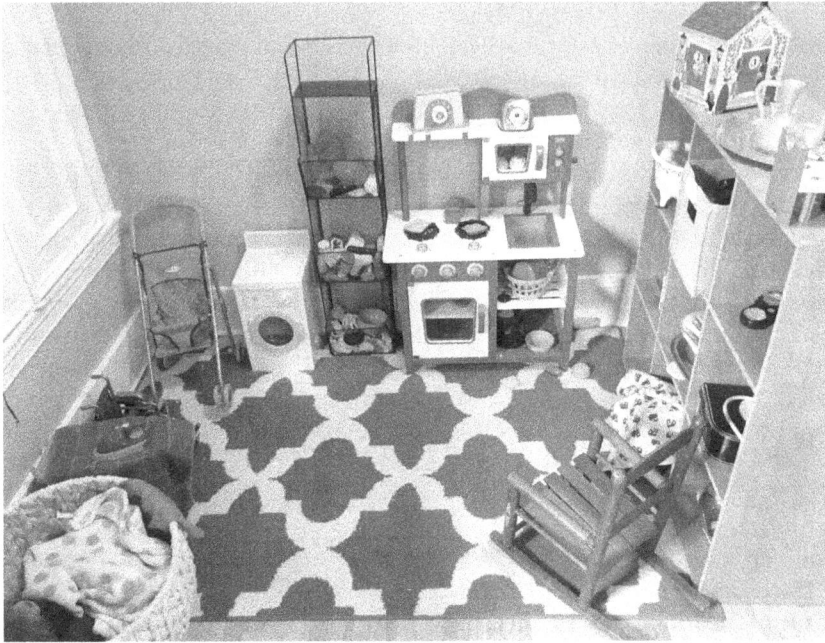

Figure 3.1 Toys that mirror the home environment.

is underdeveloped and trauma may have occurred when the child was pre-verbal, offering a linguistic narrative about a sexually abusive experience may be impossible. Many of our trauma memories are iconic and somatic, stored more in the right hemisphere of our brains than the left, experienced and stored non-linguistically, or for our youngest clients, pre-linguistically. For these children, accessing trauma narrative and allowing clients to move towards building coherence in their own stories, trauma memories take the form of glimpses and snapshots of expression in play, art or other expressive mediums. This author gives multiple clinical examples of this phenomena in other writings (Goodyear-Brown, 2019, 2019).

Expressive arts materials

Nurture House also has a fully outfitted art room that allows for a multitude of therapeutic powers to be activated through clay, paint, crafts, collage, drawing, weaving and making slime. Here the titration of materials that can access the unconscious are also offered.

Self-expression, a critically important therapeutic power of play can be fostered through expressive arts materials. Offering mediums along a continuum from most to least controllable artistic mediums can allow for children and teens to titrate their creative expressions in a safe way. To this end, instead of offering only one kind of drawing tool, like crayons, it is better to additionally offer markers, oil pastels, paint pens, coloured pencils and so forth (Landgarten, 1987).

Also, the size of space offered as a canvas for artistic expression can also serve to appropriately activate or overwhelm and shut down a child client. From postcards to large pieces of butcher paper, matching the field for expression to the containment needs of the child or teen is critical to effectively using expressive arts. Children with a sensory defensive profile may avoid clay altogether or need several options: air-dry clay, modelling clay, playdough, plasticine, in order to choose the material that fits within their window of tolerance for tactile experiences, whereas other children may glory in creating wet, slippery slime for several sessions in a row. The same is true of sand tray work. Some children will be drawn to soft Jurassic sand, others to sparkly, grainy white sand and still others to kinetic sand that is easily packed.

Sensory play

Children with all sorts of mental health issues may need regulation work to be incorporated into their therapeutic environments as well as in their academic learning environments. At Nurture House we provide a wide variety of sensory experiences aimed at meeting the child all along a continuum of their proprioceptive and vestibular needs. Some of our big body play materials are shown below. As children master big body play,

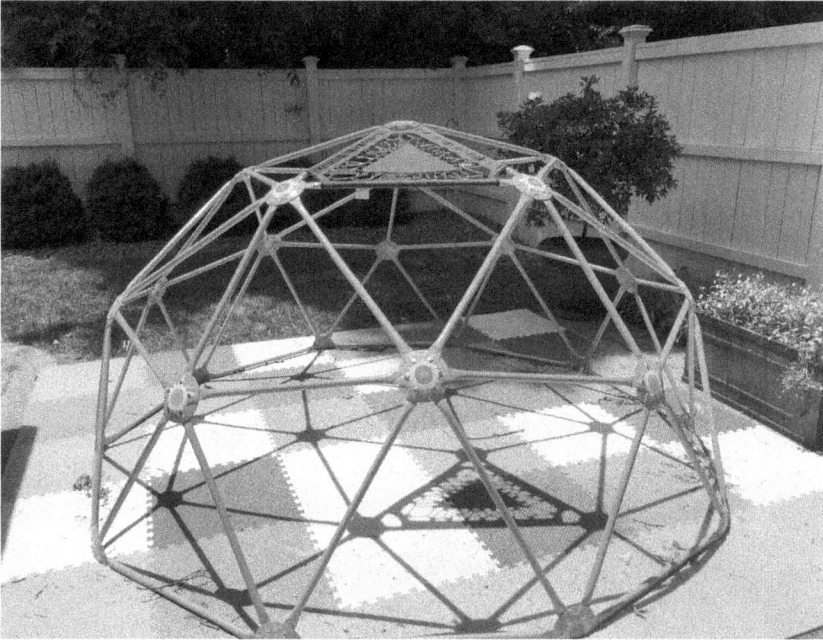

Figure 3.2 Geodome.

everything from building with giant blocks, to climbing to the top of the geodome (see Figure 3.2) and figuring out how to have a seat on top, they experience full-body mastery experiences which provide competency surges.

Creative problem solving, resiliency, self-esteem and even accelerated psychological development (four therapeutic powers of play that are all forms of increasing personal strengths) are met in this sort of play. We believe strongly in the mitigating effect of kinesthetic involvement in any kind of work that requires approaching difficult things (trauma content, eye contact, turn taking) because we have seen so many clients have break-through moments when engaged in this big body play. The jumparoo (see Figure 3.3) as well as the slackline offer big body play while enhancing attachment relationships.

We often invite a small child to stand on one side of the Jumparoo and jump as high as they can. We then invite the parent to stand on the other side and jump; without fail, the child is able to jump higher when counter weighted by the parent. This usually results in squeals of laughter and shared delight. The child who has significant trust issues due to early at-tachment wounds, who may prefer to be self-sufficient whenever possible

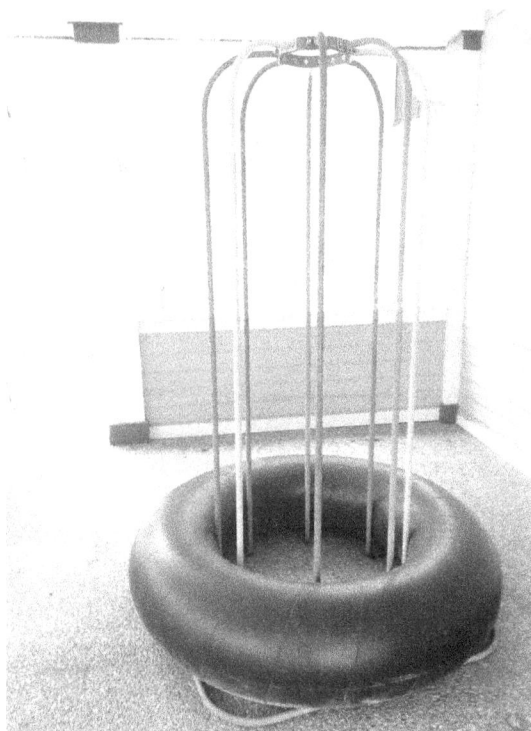

Figure 3.3 Jumparoo.

still has a strong competency urge to cross the slackline, which is impossible to do without the help of a safe other. This child is often willing to risk trusting a safe boss in small titrated doses in order to experience the eventual competency/self-esteem surge of successfully reaching the end of the slackline. The ways to incorporate attachment enhancement into this sort of big body play are almost endless.

Lastly, the somatic encoding of a state of calm can be aided by sensory play. We are grateful to have a small pool with a constantly flowing waterfall in the backyard playscape of Nurture House. While children are not allowed to swim in the pool, there are a wealth of mindfulness activities related to noticing the way their feet feel as they sit on the edge with their therapist, listening to the sound of the waterfall, experiencing the launch of worries as they sail away, and inviting them to notice what it feels like to watch something sink to the bottom. Metaphors surrounding what's on the surface and what is underneath can also be powerfully activated in preteens and adolescents through the use of this body of water.

Messy play

Children need messy play experiences, and in our scrubbed, scheduled modern world these experiences can be hard to come by, especially when the grown-ups in a child's life don't allow for mess. Play therapy spaces offer unique environments in which children can make a mess. Messy play allows for deep sensory experiences to be explored, while encouraging freedom of expression, self-regulation, positive emotions, and sometimes catharsis. Children and teens who have experienced trauma and have neurological wiring that tends towards a state of freeze or collapse, the kinaesthetic nature of messy play can often help them move out of this frozen state. Children who struggle with perfectionism also benefit from messy play as they push through the anxiety that comes from not being able to fully control the substances and become comfortable with creation not being perfect. Messy play may involve sand, water, mud puddles, playing with food (noodles, coloured rice, habitats made out of sweets). At Nurture House, we have sand trays of various sizes, including one that a child can lay down in and make snow angels. The pool and waterfall allow for much splashing and hoses, pots and dirt offer opportunities to make mud pies. The walk-in shower of the sensory room has become our messy art space. We have strung cording with clothes pins across the back wall and keep large containers of tempera paints, brushes and paper nearby. Sometimes children need the kinaesthetic experience of splattering paint. Sally, an eight-year-old survivor of sexual abuse, was having a recurring nightmare of being trapped in a room of her house with the perpetrator while the house was on fire. First she drew the bad dream scene and then she began to fling paint at the image while verbalising empowering statements about being safe now. Eventually, she got a larger brush and painted thick, long swaths of dark paints until she had covered over the image altogether.

Giving options for messy play allows children to titrate their approach to messy materials. The bathtub in the sensory room has become a ball pit and while some children benefit from the sensory experience of burying themselves underneath the balls, other children enjoy taking handfuls of balls and throwing them all around the room. With messy play of any kind it is important for the helping professional involved to have clarity about their own window of tolerance for messy play so that boundaries to the play can be established in a way that keeps the play safe for all.

How much is too much?

I recently had a child ask me, after perusing all the rooms of Nurture House and our backyard playscapes, 'do you have everything a kid needs here?' While the answer to that question is no, we do strive to provide the kinds of toys, symbols, art materials and sensory offerings that a child might need to aid in their self-expresssion. If we believe that each individual toy or sand tray miniature expands a child's vocabulary in play, wouldn't we want to offer as wide a vocabulary as we are able? The answer: not necessarily. In fact, many of the children that we see at Nurture House would be over-stimulated and experience significant dysregulation if they were brought into our dedicated sand tray room or one of our larger playrooms early on in treatment. It is a balancing act. If we only offer one cutely dressed, Caucasian baby doll in the playroom, it is unlikely that a disenfranchised child of colour, living in the inner city of Boston, would be able to identify with this doll. It is important to have figures that represent the cultural and ethnic diversity of the clients we serve. There can also be value in offering an unkempt baby doll and one who has perfectly combed hair and a per-fectly clean appearance. There is some debate about how many or how few toys should be allowed into a therapeutic playroom, and this debate gets even more heated when we dive into sand tray work. Many clinicians find themselves needing to offer both play therapy and sand tray work in the same clinical space.

Another important exploration for anyone who uses play therapeutically is whether or not broken toys are kept. Obviously, if a toy has a sharp edge or may be leaking a toxic substance, these must be discarded or repaired. Beyond that, at Nurture House we make sure that each room has some broken symbols, as we want to communicate that brokenness is allowed, perhaps even embraced, in our therapeutic spaces. We are constantly ex-panding our offerings, which begs the question, *how much is too much?*

Offering a variety of spaces, including some that are almost entirely de-void of toys, allows for therapeutic relationship, regulation and attachment to become the scaffolding upon which any other core change agents are built. I have developed a myriad of prescriptive play therapy interventions over the last 20 years. Each of these may harness a specific change agent or therapeutic power of play: direct teaching, stress management, catharsis, empathy building, attachment enhancement, etc. It would be information overload for clients if all the supplies for all these interventions were offered in one play space. To balance various therapeutic needs, we have developed a series of play spaces that are geared towards harnessing specific ther-apeutic powers of play. We have a couple of very traditional child-centred play rooms. We use these to conduct our dyadic assessments, and to engage in child-centred play therapy when this way of working is the perceived treatment need. Within each of these larger rooms, we have carved out snuggle spots that encourage containment and offer boundaried space for nurturing dyadic work. We have a small sand tray area in each of these rooms, with small sets of miniatures, but we also have a dedicated sand tray room where we often invite children to create family play genostories or create their own worlds, when they are able to navigate the stimulation of this space (see Figures 3.4 and 3.5).

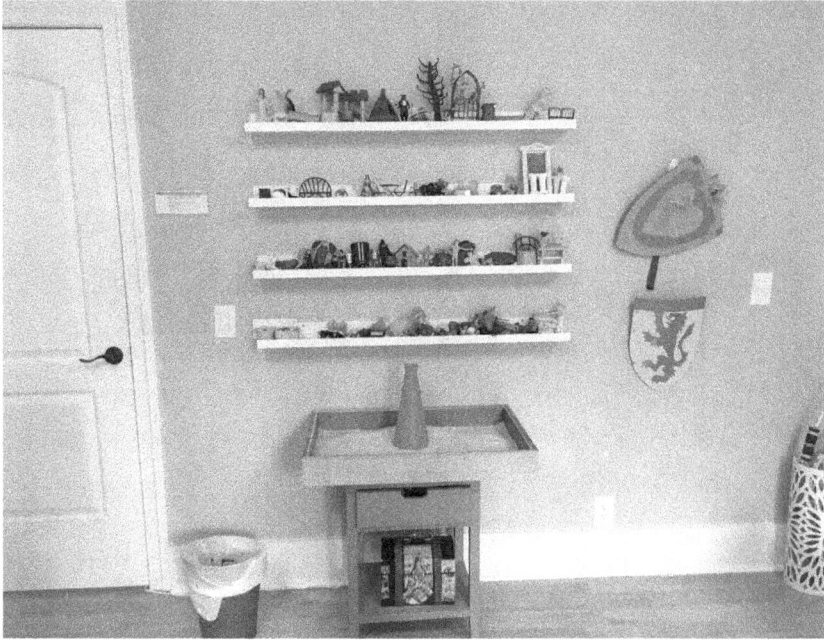

Figure 3.4 Small sand tray area.

Teens and adults often gravitate to our sand tray room for abstract symbols work. The sand tray can be a powerful tool in assessment, treatment planning, storytelling and reflective awareness work with parents. Sand tray work powerfully activates the therapeutic power of play that provides access to the unconscious. The categories of symbols/miniatures used to outfit a sand tray space is sometimes theoretically bound, but in the same way that a basic play therapy kit includes certain items, a basic kit of sand tray miniatures will include the following (while this list is not exhaustive, it will help beginning clinicians make a start): magical people (wizards and witches) and magical animals (unicorns and centaurs), domestic and wild animals, babies, helping figures, rescue vehicles, army men and army vehicles, elements of nature (stones, sticks, shells, flowers, miniature trees), jewels, furniture, fences, bridges, water, fire, scary symbols, nurturing symbols, aggressive symbols, containment devices (jails, boxes, caves, miniature handcuffs), etc. At Nurture House, we keep a small collection of symbols such as Two Face and two headed-dragons to help clients express the dichotomous nature of abusive or mentally ill caregivers. Religious symbols such as coffins, crematory vases, Buddhas, tombstones, etc. are important for all, but especially for children who are grieving.

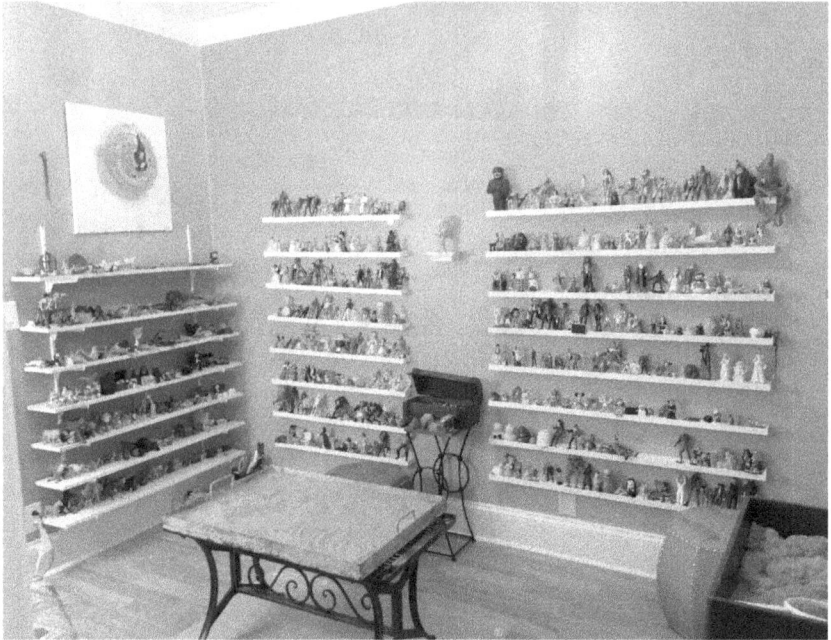

Figure 3.5 Sand tray room.

Since the relationship between the play therapist and the child is critical to therapeutic use of a play-rich environment, the number of items offered should not be overwhelming or become a distraction.

Containment

We have talked about multiple ways that containment can look within a therapeutic play space. For children with the highest distractibility or need for containment, we have developed a soothing silver-grey room with silver grey-coloured furniture in plush fabrics. The space used to be a walk-in closet with built-ins, so it is very small and immediately brings a neuro-ception of safety to many of the clients who need to feel insulated from the outside world.

Cosy rooms like this can be particularly useful when the therapist or the caregiver is the central plaything in the therapeutic process. A multitude of delighting-in games (Theraplay activities and self-created attachment en-hancement interventions) can be played in this intimate space. Materials for these games (lotion, delighting-in dice, feathers, pretend marshmallows, etc.) are kept in boxes in a neighboring room. We have a large training space in which we keep therapeutic games, our bibliotherapy library and play tools specific to particular treatment goals. We also have a whole wall of plastic boxes that offer the individual supplies needed to facilitate discrete interventions related to emotional literacy, anger management, stress inoculation, nurturing dyadic games, etc. Clinicians can choose the focussed play materials that will facilitate whatever therapeutic powers of play they are needing to activate along a continuum of treatment for an individual child, dyad or family and take it into the soothing room or another less stimulating space. When doing goal specific work, a de-stimulated environment is often most helpful. Directive play-based interventions pair positive emotion, one of the most important therapeutic powers of play, with direct or indirect teaching, problem solving, stress management or social competence. The power of the prop, whether the prop is a puppet, a magic wand, a balloon, etc., anchors the therapeutic learning while accessing all three learning portals for the child client.

Sibling groups or pull out groups of peers in classroom settings can also benefit from the therapeutic powers of play. Moral development, self-esteem, creative problem-solving, self-regulation and accelerated psychological development can all be activated through facilitated playgroup experiences. In addition to all of these change agents that increase personal strengths, many school counsellors and community mental health agencies find that the direct and indirect teaching benefits of play can be maximised in group settings. At the very least, group work allows for more children or parents to be reached at once, while normalising certain struggles that group members may share in common. Social skills training, relationship development and empathy are often activated in small group play settings. At Nurture House, we find that the strong, facilitative support of a play therapist is critical to helping children creatively solve problems related to turn taking, limit setting with one another, enhancing cooperation and overall social development when more than one child is involved. Play ranging from a shared game of pick-up sticks to two children building a block structure together, to siblings who are involved in a pretend game of cops and robbers is all rich with activation potential for the therapeutic powers of play. However, we believe that the anchoring presence of the safe boss – a helping professional who is within three to six feet (one to two meters) of the children at all times – is necessary for these powers to be activated and contained safely in therapeutic group play.

Conclusion

It is good news to children all over the world that play is being appreciated for its therapeutic benefits and incorporated into the work of many kinds of helping professionals across a myriad of clinical settings. However, being sure that we are only activating the particular therapeutic powers of play that will be most helpful to a particular child in a specific clinical circumstance requires ongoing professional development, consultation and supervision. This chapter is meant to provide a beginning template for helping professionals to use in making thoughtful decisions about the use of space and play materials in harnessing the therapeutic powers of play.

References

Bratton, S., Ray, D., Rhine, T., & Jones, L. (2005). The efficacy of play therapy with children: A meta-analytic review of treatment outcomes. *Professional Psychology: Research and Practice, 36*(4), 376–390.

Burns-Nader, S., & Hernandez-Reif, M. (2016). Facilitating play for hospitalized children through child life services. *Children's Health Care, 45*(1), 1–21.

Couch, K. J., Deitz, J. C., & Kanny, E. M. (1998). The role of play in pediatric occupational therapy. *American Journal of Occupational Therapy, 52*(2), 111–117.

De la Barra, F. (2009). Epidemiología de trastornos psiquiátricos en niños y adolescentes: Estudios de prevalencia. *Revista chilena de neuro-psiquiatría, 47*(4), 303–314.

Elkind, D. (2007). *The power of play*. Cambridge, MA: Da Capo Press.

Ginott, H. G. (1960). A rationale for selecting toys in play therapy. *Journal of Consulting Psychology, 24*, 243–246.

Goodyear-Brown, P. (2010). *Play therapy with traumatized children: A prescriptive approach*.New York: Wiley.

Goodyear-Brown, P. (2019) *Trauma and play therapy: Helping children heal*. New York. Routledge.

Goodyear-Brown, P. (2021) *Parents as Partners in Child Therapy: A Clinician's Guide*. New York. Guilford.

Green, E. J., & Christensen, T. M. (2006). Elementary school children's perceptions of play therapy in school settings. *International Journal of Play Therapy, 15*(1), 65–85.

Hall, T. M., Kaduson, H. G., & Schaefer, C. E. (2002). Fifteen effective play therapy techniques. *Professional Psychology: Research and Practice, 33*(6), 515–522.

Kessler, R. C., Berglund, P., Demler, O., Jin, R., Merikangas, K. R., & Walters, E. E. (2005). Lifetime prevalence and age-of-onset distributions of DSM-IV disorders in the National Comorbidity Survey Replication. *Archives of General Psychiatry, 62*(6), 593–602.

Kottman, T., & Meany-Walen, K. (2015). *Partners in play: An Adlerian approach to play therapy*. (3rd ed.). Alexandria, VA: American Counseling Association.

Landreth, G. L. (1993). Child-centered play therapy. *Elementary School Guidance & Counseling, 28*(1), 17–29.

Landreth, G. L. (2012). *Play therapy: The art of the relationship* (3rd ed.). New York, NY: Brunner-Routledge.

Landgarten, H. B. (1987). *Family art psychotherapy: A clinical guide and casebook*. New York: Brunner/Mazel.

Ray, D. C., Armstrong, S. A., Balkin, R. S., & Jayne, K. M. (2015). Child-centered play therapy in the schools: Review and meta-analysis. *Psychology in the Schools*, 52(2), 107–123.

Parson, J. (2017, June 18). *Puppet play therapy – Integrating theory evidence and action (ITEA)* presented at International Play Therapy Study Group. Champneys at Forest Mere, England. Adapted from Schaefer, S. C., & Drewes, A. A. (2014). *The therapeutic powers of play: 20 core agents of change* (2nd ed.). Hoboken, NJ: John Wiley.

Schaefer C. E. (1980). Play therapy. In: G. P. Sholevar, R. M. Benson, and B. J. Blinder (Eds.), *Emotional disorders in children and adolescents. Child behavior and development*. Springer: Dordrecht.

Schaefer, C. E. (1993). *The therapeutic powers of play*. Northvale, NJ: Aronson.

Schaefer, C. E., & Drewes, A. A. (2013). *The therapeutic powers of play: 20 core agents of change*. (2nd ed.). Hoboken, NJ: John Wiley & Sons.

Vygotsky, L. (1987). Thinking and speech. In L. S. Vygotsky, *Collected works* (vol. 1, pp. 39–285) (R. Rieber & A. Carton, Eds; N. Minick, Trans.). New York: Plenum.

Chapter 4

Integrating the therapeutic powers of play in nature-based settings

Maggie Fearn

Introduction

Given the opportunity, most children enjoy playing outdoors in nature. There is widespread agreement that this is to be encouraged because in natural environments they can develop confidence and independence. Children can encounter species other than their own and explore environments that expand their awareness and tolerance of a broad range of sensory experiences, supporting resilience. They can test their ability and come up with creative solutions. Playing outdoors accelerates development; children learn from trial and error and risk taking, and they develop both social skills and a strong sense of self (Hanscom, 2016; Moss, 2012; Play Wales, 2015). Most parents and grandparents remember playing freely outdoors when they were children. They share fond memories of 'playing out' for hours, having adventurous moments alone or with friends, away from the adult gaze, coming home in the twilight, dirty, tired, hungry and smiling. These play memories tend to be nostalgic, and many of these same parents will say that their own children's access to playing out is restricted. For many families there are significant barriers including increasing urbanisation, privatisation of open spaces, cramped living spaces, environmental degradation, risk aversion, time poverty and lack of affordable transport, all impacting severely on access to and enjoyment of play in nature in the world beyond the home for all but the lucky few (Louv, 2010; Natural England, 2009; RSPB Cymru, 2012).

For many years education and play providers in Europe and USA have made considerable effort to proactively counteract this world view, spearheaded by influential advocates who provide evidence that contact with nature enhances well-being (Hanscom, 2016; Louv, 2010; Maller, Townsend, Pryor, Brown, and St Leger 2006, March). Some enlightened authorities support the creation of small pockets of natural regeneration, oases of wildness in school grounds and parks, providing natural spaces for children to play within their own neighbourhoods (Gill, 2011). As well as providing access to the benefits of playing in nature, these initiatives are developing the next generation of naturalists. Early contact with nature through direct experience is considered vital in encouraging positive and proactive environ-mental values and behaviours (Frazier, 2019; Natural England, 2009). Children who play in nature tend to grow up loving and protective of nature, which supports the development of compassionate and altruistic traits (Gibson, 1979; Wilson, 1986). However, existential anxiety about the impact of man-made global warming and climate change creates a sense of respon-sibility for nature that can be overwhelming. It is evident that, to survive, more-than-human nature needs our awareness and advocacy equally as much as we need access to nature for our mental and physical health (Macy & Young Brown, 2014). Ultimately, both human and non-human survival de-pends on this dynamic relationship (Seymour, 2016; Suzuki, 1999). Practitioners concerned with child and adolescent mental health need to be aware of this ambivalent and complex reality. If we are to draw on the healing powers of nature, we must also be prepared to create spaces in which nature can regenerate, otherwise we are colluding in its exploitation and passing on our responsibilities as adults to children and young people.

Nature-based interventions for supporting mental health focus on the power of nature for connection, inspiration, healing and support, providing an en-vironment that is both backdrop to therapist/client relationship, and supplier of experiences (Berger and McLeod, 2006; Chown, 2014). There is a parallel thesis that places the 'ecological self' in connection with the cycles and rhythms of nature, and this links with the importance of continuity and meaning in the rituals of tradition, culture and religion, creating narratives and dramatic me-taphors that resonate with traumatised clients (Goodyear-Brown, 2018; Totton, 2011). It is also proposed that working therapeutically with groups and individuals in the outdoors involves the natural environment as a significant presence in building a therapeutic relationship, and it is a necessary prerequisite for sensory-motor integration (Fearn, 2014; Goodyear-Brown, 2018).

Kestly (2014) conceptualises the safety of therapeutic relationship in a spatial dimension. She explores the relationship between play therapist and child as a form of sanctuary, defined as a psychological space that provides safety, refuge and protection in which to pursue a special need without fear of intrusion, criticism or predation. A sanctuary can also be a physical space for quiet at-tention, acceptance and open heartedness, often associated with wildlife con-servation and worship. Kalff proposes that one of the primary tasks of sandplay therapy is to provide the child with the experience of 'a free and protected space for emotional healing' (Kalff, 2003, p. 17). Introducing a child to the sand box in therapy provides a miniaturised and projected world in the context of all-encompassing psychological containment of therapeutic relationship, and invites the child into an imaginative space where it is safe to re-organise and make sense of traumatic experience through play in the sanctuary of therapeutic relationship (Lowenfeld, 2005). In play therapy this re-organisation occurs deep in the physiology of the body through playful relationship, trans-forming the traumatised nervous system's default anticipation of threat to an expectation of safety, which leads to increasingly satisfying and fun experiences through the sensory and perceptive medium of play (Gaskill & Perry, 2014). The child's inner world of sensing, perceiving and anticipating is brought into balance through interaction with a rich play environment through playful activity. There is a meeting of worlds at the boundary of the skin (Fearn & Troccoli, 2017).

When considering applying this understanding to nature-based play therapy, we can see that Lowenfeld's (2005) and Kalff's (2003) ideas of miniaturised invitational space resonates with affordance theory (Fjørtoft, 2001; Gibson, 1979; Kyttä, 2002). The theory of affordances seeks to define how the natural environment offers opportunities for human interaction and immersion, resulting in systemic change. The author's experience of developing marginal woodland edges into playspaces for children over a ten-year period provides a living example of this dynamic relationship between child and nature. Spontaneous, unplanned play activity moves children freely through the space and the space shapeshifts in response to the children's play. Wildlife, trees, plants, soil and air inhabit the space alongside, beneath and within the playing children, offering invitations to climb, run, build, hide, slide, dig, discover, shriek, call, whisper and be still (Fearn, 2014; North and Fearn, 2010). The natural environment is the provider of the sensory-motor cues for interactive, intersubjective play, and intrasubjective developmental growth occurs.

Informed by early childhood education and care research into outdoor play environments, Kernan (2010) proposes that 'the outdoors' encompasses three interconnecting fields, or arenas of action. These are described as indoor-outdoor connectedness, the enclosed outdoor space and the wider outdoors. 'Indoor-outdoor connectedness' suggests that, while indoors, children are able to perceive affordances for action outdoors, and to be touched by different qualities of light and sound. The semi-permeable boundary of glass and transitional spaces allows sensory information and cues for action to enter the indoor space. Attention to design of the transition points between indoors and outdoors creates invitations, for example vistas through windows and entrances and exits through arches and doorways. This eases movement between indoors and outdoors, making it possible to bring the outdoors in and the indoors outside, actually and imaginatively. If a child responds to the invitations, 'the enclosed outdoor space' offers the availability of potential affordances for action, exploration and play for different ages, stages of development, interests and abilities. This accords to the amount of space available and the surface layout with naturally occurring and designed features such as different levels, slopes, steps, platforms, pathways, routes and small spaces, hidey holes, dens, nature elements and plant and animal life. Imaginative play is encouraged by the availability of 'loose parts' and transformable materials (Nicholson, 1971). Attention is paid to the degree of comfort for children and adults, including compass orientation and sun path, shelter, seating and provision of opportunities to swing, climb, roll, run and rest (Fearn, 2014). Kernan (2010) designates 'the wider outdoors' for unsupervised play, where children can pass through their neighbourhood beyond the 'enclosed outdoor space', exploring green spaces, parks, wilderness, and other public and community spaces that contain a range of physical features and potential for social contact. All three domains are influenced by the availability of affordances and the extent to which they are perceived, utilised or shaped by children, and promoted or constrained by adults.

This chapter proposes that nature-based play therapy utilises indoor-outdoor connectedness and the enclosed outdoor space, expanding the psychological and intersubjective sanctuary of therapeutic relationship into the physical sanctuary of nature as an extension of the play therapy room.

The case studies

The nature-based therapeutic setting for these case studies has been designed using the principles set out above. The playroom has a French window that opens onto a covered veranda, and a small garden, with a woodland edge and the sound of a stream and waterfall beyond. There is a fire pit in the garden, raised decking and a quiet area near the waterfall with a hammock. We can sling a slack rope between two trees, and the garden is on different levels with a pathway winding intriguingly into the woods.

Both case studies involve children who experienced early paediatric medical trauma, and have developed unique strategies to cope with the impact of a bewildering world on immature nervous systems. Both children have loving parents who want the best for their child. Significant details have been changed to protect their identity and only relevant details of their play have been included.

Indoor-outdoor connectedness and the therapeutic powers of play

Jodie was aged six years at the time of referral. She is a lively, popular and intelligent child who, since birth, has very limited movement and feeling in her lower body. From infancy onwards she endured several invasive medical procedures. In her referral, Jodie's mother described how Jodie struggled with frustration at the high level of care she needs, expressing a longing for more independence. Considerable pent-up aggressive energy made her reactive. She turned this energy on her loving parents and in on herself and had extreme rages followed by long periods of sadness and depression. We agreed to 15 sessions of play therapy, beginning in the play therapy room with an introduction to the outdoors area. On her first visit, Jodie had been out onto the veranda with her mother, from where she had seen into the garden and heard the stream, but she did not ask to go any further and soon returned indoors.

Because of her care needs, her mother accompanied Jodie to play therapy. She was a sensitive, reassuring presence, a fascinated witness to the developing therapeutic relationship between the play therapist and her daughter. As therapy progressed she was also drawn into the play by Jodie and given challenging roles that deepened her understanding of Jodie's lived experience and their relationship.

At first there were several sensory play sessions in which Jodie uses the materials to express her messy mixed up feelings, mixing flour, water and food colouring into 'disgusting messes' (her word) that overflow the bowl and spread uncontrollably. Gradually she thickens the mixture and keeps it in the container. As her sensory play becomes calmer and more contained, we glimpse episodes from her lived experience of medical trauma in brief, projective miniaturised play in the sand box. This intense, anxious play is repeated at the beginning of the next two sessions, followed by sensory, regulatory activity. She makes sticky dough, which gradually becomes drier and easier to shape into imaginative forms, and this leads to her preference for clay and a corresponding expansion of awareness and response to her environment. The following describes two sessions mid-way through therapy.

As the intensity of her play in the sand box subsides, she creates form from the clay. She makes a fish and a carrot, and this develops into a fishing game with a ball of string and the carrot as bait to catch the fish. She instructs the play therapist and her mother to carry her to 'the pond' (her word). She indicates in the direction of the stream, which is 20 metres across the garden and into the woods. When we get there she leaves her fishing line, bait and catch hanging over the stream and she asks to come straight back into the play therapy room.

At the start of the next session she tells several quick stories in the sand box, returning to previous themes but without the intensity of feeling. She then makes a loaf of bread with kinetic sand and she says 'Let's play differently today'. She requests that we all go back to 'the pond' and this time we stay there for most of the session. Jodie throws her line into the stream and pulls it back over and over again, 'fishing' she says. Then we cross the stream and she wraps hazel leaves in a knotted cloth, 'for tea with the loaf'. 'It is time to go home', she says and she ties one end of the ball of string to a tree by the stream and unrolls the ball all the way back 20 metres to the veranda and sits holding the string, with her mother beside her. She then sends the play therapist back along the string to the stream, and for the remaining few minutes of the session we communicate with each other by tugs on the line, back and forth across her expanded play territory.

This session was a turning point in Jodie's therapeutic journey. Her mother reported that she was often sunny and positive at home, and her teacher noticed how much more engaged she was. In play therapy she made full use of the play therapy room to challenge herself physically, asking for help when she needed. She immersed herself in imaginative play involving her mother and the play therapist. She did not return to the stream again, however her play was expansive and included imaginary journeys and maps. For her final session she requested that we cook sausages in the garden, and we ate them on the veranda, enjoying the liminal space between indoors and out.

This case study demonstrates how, through the medium of sensory play, and in the safety of relationship with her mother and the play therapist, Jodie was able to express her difficult feelings, find support and regulate herself. Then, using the miniaturised sanctuary of the sand box and the 'as if' safety of symbolic play, she was able to play out her traumatic pre-verbal experiences. This reorganisation of her internal world and increasing sense of coherence and predictability enabled her attention to shift from survival mode and to perceive the affordances of her environment. She could access the support she needed to actively and creatively respond to the cues from indoor-outdoor connectedness. This offered her the opportunity for seamless extension and expansion within the metaphor of play. Through play she expanded her imaginative territory into the enclosed outdoor space and she manifested a symbol of connection and communication that so vividly resonated with her experience of therapeutic relationship with her mother and the play therapist.

The enclosed outdoor space and the therapeutic powers of play

Ben, aged 13, was referred by his mother because of her concerns for his well-being. She described high levels of anxiety. In exploring his developmental history, she told me he had experienced a difficult Caesarean section birth and was immediately separated from her in intensive care. She mentioned that he had always found transitions very stressful and that he was severely affected by a recent emotional upset in the family. She described how he shut down into a defensive, dissociated state, and often complained of terrible headaches and nausea. He found school very challenging and often begged to stay at home or needed picking up early. As Ben entered adolescence, he was unsure of himself and found social life confusing. Home was very important to him and he was comfortable both indoors and out. He spent time on a screen indoors, he liked being with his family and he was confident being outdoors, walking and cycling miles on his own in the neighbouring countryside. He gave the impression of unreachable insularity, to those who did not know him well, and showed warm caring humour with those whom he trusted. It was evident it would take some time for him to establish a trusting relationship with a therapist. We agreed on 20 sessions with the option of nature-based play therapy.

From the start of therapy he prefers to be outside, he leads the way and I follow, staying within the metaphors of his play, paying careful attention to my use of self, particularly in relation to how I approach him, where I stand in relation to him, how I mirror his non-verbal responses and noticing my own comfort levels. As our relationship develops, Ben gradually includes me in his world, and I am able to respond proactively to themes and follow the threads of his play. In the first two sessions he builds piles of stones along the pathway to the woods, which he says are like the stone cairns he has seen on the moorland. The next session he makes a figure out of deadwood and a small animal skull that he found and stands it at the entrance to the woods as the guardian. He seems to be marking the boundaries of the therapeutic space with his own protective symbols, and I sense that together we are starting out on a journey to find his true self, working from the outside inwards, responsive to sensory play cues from the natural environment.

We make a hearth in the woods, a place to sit by and return to, where Ben creates a ritual of making a fire in a stick stove, collecting and feeding it with kindling, and dousing it, to poke the wet ashes with a long stick. One day he draws a line on the ground with the ash tipped stick and I suggest he draws a circle around himself and imagines it as a boundary to keep out whatever he does not want. I ask him to imagine what his boundary is made of and he need not tell me what that is. I want him to experience making a choice about whether to share his thoughts. Then I suggest he search for found objects to symbolise what he wants to keep inside his boundary. In this way he begins to define his personal space using the circle, a symbol of wholeness (Kalff, 2003), and he gets to decide what he wants to keep close and what he wants to keep away. Working at the stick fire afterwards, he remarks on the exact distance that he can feel the heat of the flames on his skin, and he says that would be what the monsters would feel if they got too close to his boundary. Staying in the safety of the metaphor of imaginative play he communicates how he is gaining control over his innermost fears.

I usually keep time and tell him when we have five minutes left to the end of each session. One session he decides we do it together without a watch, to practise sensing time passing. I find this quite challenging, having to let go of controlling the session's time limit, while he is relaxed and remarkably accurate. I am witnessing his wakening perceptions and increasing sense of personal control and noticing how this affects our relationship. As he gains self-possession, he trusts me enough to close his eyes to count by feel the acorns and hazelnuts I place in the palm of his hand, then he roasts them, we taste them and compare them, finding language to accurately describe their different tastes and smells. Through playing with his senses, he becomes more confident and he risks stepping into a new unknown, exploring his sense of balance, and playing with his fear of heights. He climbs a tree, he lies in a rocking hammock taking both feet off the ground and he balances on a slack rope, using a long walking stick on one side and my hand on the other, then two long walking sticks, then one balance pole.

His inward gaze moves outwards to support his balance, his proprioceptive sense defines his orientation in space. This is a very important shift, because he is no longer caught in the anxious grip of fearful anticipation that takes him away from the present moment. Instead he is calm and minutely responsive to environmental feedback through all his senses.

Over time he begins to express difficult feelings that have been so long buried beneath somatic symptoms of migraines and nausea. With support, he practises moving through frustration and anger. We stomp around the fire, he finds his voice, calling out and swearing lustily. Finally, he douses the fire with a whole bucket of water, and bursts out laughing. I witness this release of long held pain and how he shifts into fluid, joyful movement. It is exhilarating. Another day, I notice how his immersion in sensory play comes with a felt sense of deep satisfaction. He melts beeswax in a pot on the fire and mixes it with ash, soil, and leaves. He manipulates the warm wax mixture, his whole hand coated like a second skin, and when it cools he peels it off. It reminds me of the protective vernix on a newborn baby and conjures metaphors of rebirth and renewal.

Playing in nature and with natural materials and elements, Ben defines his outermost boundaries and then, moving inwards he finds his way back in time to his earliest felt-sense memories. Responding to the feedback loop between inner and outer worlds he changes from being without boundaries, to meeting the outside world at the boundary of his skin. He is able to differentiate how he receives and responds to sensory information from the environment and how he feels, moves and senses within his body. By naming this, finding language for perception, he can stay present and he dissociates less often. This ability to sustain engagement and joint attention leads to strengthening peer friendships, and his experience of school becomes more positive. His teachers report a significant change in his ability to engage with learning. He is re-assessed as developmentally on track and he is referred to specialist help for dyslexia.

Conclusion

These case studies demonstrate how the richness of nature-based play therapy affords enhanced opportunities for accessing core agents of change inherent in the therapeutic powers of play. Both children were able to express their unconscious feelings and make sense of their experiences through playing imaginatively in nature. Playing in and with the natural environment, they were able to benefit from therapeutic relationship. They were able to self-regulate, benefitting from sensory and perceptive feedback that supports them to be present and alive in the moment. Both case studies highlight the individual child's remarkable drive to self-heal, given the necessary conditions to do so. Many factors contribute to a child's recovery in nature-based play therapy, including a multi-sensory environment that offers opportunities for developmentally appropriate play, caring attention, sensitive timing and astute responsiveness. The case examples show that a child experiences a nature-based therapeutic space as a seamless extension of the play therapy room: a boundaried, protecting, safe space that offers opportunities for immersion in the therapeutic powers of playing in and with nature, indoors and out. This protective experience supports the child and equips them for the challenges of their lived world in the wider outdoors beyond the sanctuary of nature-based play therapy.

References

Berger, R. & McLeod, J. (2006). Incorporating nature into therapy: A framework for practice. *Journal of Systemic Therapies*, *25*, 80–94.

Chown, A. (2014). *Play therapy in the outdoors: Taking play therapy out of the playroom and into natural environments*. London: Jessica Kingsley Publishers.

Fjørtoft, I. (2001). The natural environment as a playground for children: The impact of outdoor play activities in pre-primary school children. *Early Childhood Education Journal*, *29*(2), 111–117.

Fearn, M. (2014). Working therapeutically with groups in the outdoors: A natural space for healing. In E. Prendiville & J. Howard (Eds.), *Play therapy today*. Oxon: Routledge.

Fearn, M. & Troccoli, P. (2017). Being, becoming and healing through movement and touch. In E. Prendiville & J. Howard (Eds.), *Creative psychotherapy: Applying the principles of neurobiology to play and expressive arts-based therapies*. Oxon: Routledge.

Frazier, N. (2019). *How to raise an outdoors kid*. The New Nature Movement: Children and Nature Network. Retrieved 02.11.19 from https://www.childrenandnature.org/2019/01/31/how-to-raise-an-outdoors-kid-tips-to-jump-start-a-childhood-outdoors.

Gaskill, R. L. & Perry, B. D. (2014). The neurobiological power of play. In C. Malchiodi & D. Crenshaw (Eds.), *Creative arts and play therapy for attachment problems*. New York: The Guilford Press.

Gibson, J. J. (1979). *The ecological approach to visual perception*. Boston: Houghton-Mifflin.

Gill, T. (2011). *Sowing the seeds: Reconnecting London's children with nature*. London: Greater London Authority (London Sustainable Development Commission).

Goodyear Brown, P. (2019). *Trauma and play therapy. Helping children heal*. New York: Routledge.

Hanscom, A. J. (2016). *Balanced and barefoot*. Oakland, CA: New Harbinger Publications Inc.

Kalff, D. (2003). *Sandplay: A psychotherapeutic approach to the psyche*. Cloverdale, CA: Temenos Press. (Original work published 1980).

Kernan, M. (2010). Outdoor affordances in early childhood education and care settings: Adults' and children's perspectives. *Children, Youth and Environments*, *20*(1), 152–177.

Kestly, T. A. (2014). *The interpersonal neurobiology of play: Brain building interventions for emotional well-being*. New York: W.W. Norton & Company.

Kyttä, M. (2002). Affordances of children's environments in the context of cities, small towns, suburbs and rural villages in Finland and Belarus. *Journal of Environmental Psychology*, 22, 109–123.

Louv, R. (2010). *Last child in the woods: Saving our children from nature-deficit disorder*. USA: Atlantic Books.

Lowenfeld, M. (2005). *Understanding children's sandplay: Lowenfeld's world technique*. UK: Sussex Academic Press.

Macy, J. & Young Brown, M. (2014). *Coming back to life*. Canada: New Society Publishers.

Maller, C., Townsend, M., Pryor, A., Brown, P. & St Leger, L. (2006, March). Healthy nature healthy people: 'contact with nature' as an upstream health promotion intervention for populations. *Health Promotion International*, 21(1), 45–54.

Moss, S. (2012). *Natural childhood*. UK: National Trust Report.

Natural England. (2009). *Childhood and nature: A survey on changing relationships with nature across generations*. Cambridge, UK: Natural England. Retrieved 05.11.19 from http://publications.naturalengland.org.uk/publication/5853658314964992.

Nicholson, S. (1971). How not to cheat children: The theory of loose parts. *Landscape Architecture*, 62, 30–34.

North, S., & Fearn, M. (2010). Validating child led play in the context of forest school: Play based pedagogy and children's perspectives. Unpublished. Paper presented at *FCW conference Cardiff*, November 2010 and IOL UK Forest School Conference, October 2011. PDF available: Movement Sense cic. info@movementsense.co.uk.

Play Wales. (2015). *Playing out and about. Play for Wales, Spring* (issue 44), 8–11.

RSPB Cymru. (2012). *Every child outdoors wales*. Wales: RSPB.

Seymour, V. (2016). The human-nature relationship and its impact on health: A critical review. *Frontiers of Public Health*, 4, 260.

Suzuki, D. (1999). *The sacred balance: Rediscovering our place in nature*. B.C. Canada: Greystone Books.

Totton, N. (2011). *Wild therapy: Undomesticating inner and outer worlds*. Ross on Wye: PCCS Books.

Wilson, E. O. (1986). *Biophilia. The human bond with other species*. Cambridge USA: Harvard Publishing.

Part II

Travelling through the continents

Embodiment-Projection-Role sequence

Travelling through the Embodiment-Projective-Role continents, you will meet Christopher, Amber, Jonathon and Sally, and their gifted therapists, as we navigate the developmental stages linking play and the achievement of physical, emotional, and social identity. Christopher's sensory play provides the route to self-regulation; Amber uses small world play to find safety and gain empowerment over difficult emotions; Jonathon finally learns to play and Sally finds her Self through elaborate role play scenarios.

Chapter 5

Calming Christopher

The regulating powers of sensory play

Siobhán Prendiville

Introduction to sensory play

Usher (2010, p. 2) defines sensory play as 'play that provides opportunities for children and young people to use all their senses, or opportunities to focus play to encourage the use of one particular sense'. Gascoyne (2011, p. 2) proposes that it is the sensory focus of sensory play that 'adds a significant and integral extra dimension to the play', which differentiates it from other types of play. She also suggests that most play 'has the potential to be sensory' as play in itself engages the senses (2011, p. 2). Essentially, sensory play involves using the body to experience the world through the senses: touch, smell, taste, sight, hearing and movement. It is play that engages one, many or all of the sensory systems: visual, auditory, tactile, olfactory, gustatory, vestibular, proprioceptive and interoceptive (Prendiville & Fearn, 2017, pp. 121–122). Prendiville (2021) explores and defines sensory play therapy, proposing that sensory play therapy intentionally uses sensory play to activate the therapeutic powers of play.

The body, and moving the body, are central in sensory play. Jennings (1999) defines this type of play, which incorporates body movement, as 'embodiment play'. Jennings' pivotal focus on the body as the primary means of learning, and the critical importance of sensory play, are evident in both her neuro-dramatic play and developmental playtherapy model, also referred to as embodiment-projective-role. Embodiment play focusses on primary physicalised experiences, which are predominantly expressed through the senses and body movement. Large and small body movements, dancing, chanting, exploration and interaction and rhythmic and sensory play take prominence during the embodiment stage. This type of play is essential in the development of physical identity (Jennings, 1999, 2011).

The importance of incorporating sensory play in therapeutic work with children and families also features strongly in Brody's developmental play therapy (Brody, 1978, 1993), dynamic play therapy (Harvey, 1994, 2008), and Theraplay® (Booth & Jernberg, 2010). Each of these established therapies clearly emphasise the curative power of touch and the profound

therapeutic value of sensory play including physical play, rhythmic movement, playful body contact games and nurturing touch. The focus on sensory play in these therapies is grounded in attachment theory and has been
validated from a neurodevelopmental perspective (Prendiville, 2021).

Sensory play provides developmentally and neurobiologically appropriate opportunities to discern internal and external conditions and experiences, process sensory information, gain understanding of what is going
on and respond within a comfortable range of arousal (Prendiville & Fearn,
2017, pp. 121–122). Somatosensory play holds many potential benefits for
children, teenagers and adults. It is fun and engaging (Beckerleg, 2009;
Gascoyne, 2011), it absorbs the player (Fearn, 2014, p. 116) and it is a
significant source of joy for our brain (Panksepp, 1998). Sensory play
promotes sensory integration (Godwin Emmons & McKendry Anderson,
2005), facilitates psychological development (Prendiville, S., 2014), promotes play development (Jennings, 1999; Stagnitti, 1998, 2009) and supports the development of attachment (Cozolino, 2010; Nelson, 2008;
Schore, 2005; Schore & Schore, 2008). Rhythmic, repetitive, patterned
somatosensory play experiences are necessary to activate and supply or-
ganising neural input to the brainstem and the mid-brain (Bruce, 2011;
Perry, 2006). The ability of sensory play to both soothe and stimulate the
nervous system is key in its ability to successfully treat persistent nervous
system reactivity to trauma and stress (Prendiville & Fearn, 2017).

The case study provided in this chapter illustrates the integration of core
sensory play activities and techniques in a child's psychotherapy process. It
highlights the power of sensory play in evoking therapeutic and life-long
changes. The discussion that follows the case study aims to bring the
therapeutic powers of sensory play to life by clearly identifying the specific
change agents that were activated through sensory play in the case study.

Introduction to the central client

Christopher, aged 6.5 years, was referred for play therapy by his parents. At
the time of referral he was experiencing severe difficulties at home, in school
and during other organised activities. He was described by his parents as
being extremely angry, having multiple daily outbursts and meltdowns
where he would scream, kick, hit and bite others. In addition, both his
parents and his teacher described him as being very impulsive and ex-
hibiting acute difficulties with attention, concentration and listening. Poor
social skills were also identified, his teacher described him as being isolated
in school. At the time of referral Christopher had no friends. It was also
reported that he told many lies, often cursed at others and regularly shouted
at people instead of talking to them. Food and feeding were also identified
as an ongoing difficulty. Christopher ate a very limited repertoire of food,
mealtimes at home were very stressful. His parents wanted Christopher to

sit at the dining table for meals; instead he would run around the table, climb the couches and jump on furniture. His father would often have to spoon feed him in order to get him to ingest any food. Christopher's mother had disengaged from meal times as she found them too stressful.

Christopher spent the first two years of his life in an orphanage. His biological mother had severe drug and alcohol problems, and she abandoned him when he was two months old. Video footage from the orphanage showed him as silent and withdrawn. He sat alone and did not attempt to interact with staff members or other infants in the setting. His parents reported that he had no words or vocalisations when they adopted him and that he did not cry until he had been with them over six months. At the time of referral Christopher was living in a rural area with both his parents. He did not have any siblings, he did have some contact with cousins of similar age; however, he did not engage in joint play when with them. He often disrupted their play and displayed aggressive behaviours towards them.

Case study illustrating the integration of the therapeutic powers of sensory play

The therapist conducted intake sessions with Christopher's parents and his current teacher. School reports from previous years indicated that the presenting issues had been evident since Christopher started preschool. Christopher's parents and teacher completed Goodman's (1997) strengths and difficulties questionnaires (SDQ) both of whom placed Christopher in the abnormal category for each area: emotional problems, conduct problems, hyperactivity, peer problems and pro-social. Christopher did not have a formal diagnosis at the time of referral, it was suggested that he should attend psychotherapy using play therapy before any diagnostic assessment was carried out. Having completed intake sessions the therapist created a *Therapeutic Touchstone* story (Prendiville, 2014b) for Christopher. She told Christopher this story in the first session with him; his parents were present for the storytelling. She then continued into a child-centred play therapy approach (Landreth, 2012) in order to attempt to build a relationship with Christopher and assess how to proceed with the therapy.

During the initial child-centred play therapy sessions, Christopher presented as chaotic, he was extremely busy in the room moving from play material to play material, picking things up, looking at them, mouthing some and throwing them onto the ground. He needed to leave the playroom frequently to check in on his parents in the waiting room; when he did so he would cling to his mother, she would offer comforting words, but he would remain dysregulated. His play was totally chaotic and disorganised, he did not demonstrate any imaginative play skills and was unable to engage in any sustained play, other than with the fidget box and sensory play materials. The only play materials that held his attention were the sensory ones. During his second session Christopher engaged with the sensory box for 20 minutes, feeling, squeezing, stretching, looking at, bouncing and rubbing the various fidget and sensory toys. He also engaged in bubble blowing repeatedly during the first three sessions.

After three sessions with Christopher the therapist further developed her case formulation. A number of key factors guided the therapist's decision making: it was clear that Christopher had extreme regulation difficulties and poor play skills, he found it difficult to be away from his parents for sustained periods of time, the comfort and support his parents offered him was not actually regulating for him and Christopher was drawn to the sensory play materials available in the therapy room. With these in mind the therapist decided to move forward in the following ways:

1   meet Christopher's parents for a review session and also complete some sensory play and relational play with them.
2   through regular parent sessions she would support Christopher's parents to build daily sensory play experiences into home life. They would focus on physical play activities, parent-child relational play and regulatory play with fidgets and sensory materials.
3   include parent-child relational play at the beginning and end of each of Christopher's play therapy sessions.
4   alter the playroom to better suit Christopher's current developmental level. The therapist wanted to ensure that the playroom afforded opportunities for as much sensory play as possible. Space and appropriate sensory play materials were essential. For Christopher's sessions, the therapist removed many of the projective and role play materials, board games and toys with small pieces. She brought in a wider array of sensory materials including coloured rice, lentils, pasta, coloured sand, water, water beads, bubble bath, baby lotion, flour, cornflour etc., rattles, soft blankets, soothers and baby bottles. A tent, tunnel and exercise balls were more prominent in the room now that many of the other play materials were removed.
5   move from child-centred play therapy (Landreth, 2012) techniques into more interactive sensory play therapy techniques (Prendiville, 2021) in her 1:1 work with Christopher.
6   as the therapist developed more insight into the types of sensory play that were regulating for Christopher she would link in with his school and support them in incorporating daily sensory play rituals for Christopher.

The parent-child relational play and Theraplay® activities were challenging to manage initially. The therapist remained regulated, focussed and playful and she kept the play activities physical and short. When Christopher discovered that the games were based on sensory interaction and were fun he soon began to join in easily and really enjoyed the special time with his parents. There were some sensations that Christopher could not tolerate initially, certain touches, e.g. cotton ball touch, and he could not lie down for any physical games. He also could not accept food directly from the therapist or either of his parents. He was never coerced into any of these, instead the therapist reflected his discomfort and suggested alternative sensory play-based games.

Physical and rhythmic games such as row your boat, piggyback rides, horsey games and wheelbarrow walks brought laughter, touch and connection. Cradling, cuddling and rocking soon followed. Bubble and ball games, simple feather touching games, making up special handshakes and mirroring and copying games soon became firm favourites also. *Simon Says*, *Traffic Light* and *Mother May I?* games also began to enter the room. While initially Christopher could not lie on the ground, he soon began to love being pulled around the room in a blanket. After time this moved into him being swung in a blanket while his Mum or Dad sang him a very special song about how loved and safe he is. Massage, *Peek a Boo* and *Hide and Seek* were some of the final games to emerge in our parent-child relational play; at first Christopher was unable to play any of these, over time they brought him the most delight.

For 16 sessions, the parent and child relational play sessions framed the therapist's 1:1 interactive sensory play sessions (Prendiville, 2021) with Christopher. During these sessions the aim was to facilitate therapeutic alliance and connection, to enrich and develop Christopher's play skills and also to establish the types of sensory input that were soothing and stimulating for Christopher. The therapist became more directive in her interactions, she introduced physical games, dancing, singing and rhythmical movement. She made silly faces, introduced and played with simple attention grabber toys such as a glove puppet, bubbles, balloons and party blowers. This began to hold Christopher's attention; he started to laugh and join in the play with the therapist. As time passed, he began to take the lead in the games, initiating play ideas in the sessions. He loved exploring the sensory play materials, initially he was drawn to dry materials such as the coloured rice, lentils and dry sand, but he quickly moved into wet messier materials also. He fully engaged with the materials, feeling them, licking and tasting some of the edible ones. The therapist modelled sprinkling these materials over her arm, scooping them up, transferring them into different containers, shaping and moulding them. Christopher began to copy and then extend the play. The therapist began adding sound effects and gestures to his play. Christopher began transferring the materials from one container to another, listening to the sounds they made, and gradually began to mix some together and explore what happened when he did. He soon figured out how to pour just the right amount of water in so that it wouldn't overflow! He started to engage in water play for sustained periods of time, he loved adding in different smells, immersing his hands and arms in the water. He thoroughly enjoyed it when the therapist dried his hands and rubbed hand cream in them. Soon little cars and figures made their way into the sand and other dry materials. The baby doll found her way into the water. Christopher's play was expanding into the projective realm. By session 13 Christopher's play was calm, relaxed and organised. In this session he spent time playing with the sensory materials, moved into exploring instruments and continued into play with playdough and finger painting. As Christopher's play expanded, the less intrusive the therapist became (Yasenik & Gardner, 2012). She began to make more use of tracking and reflecting commentary, she noticed and recognised achievements and efforts. Throughout these sessions Christopher also spent a great deal of time engaging in self-directed regulatory play with fidget toys and other sensory materials.

As these sessions progressed the therapist made further recommendations to Christopher's teachers and parents about appropriate sensory play and regulating activities to use with Christopher. As the lower brain learns by repetition, she felt it was crucial that Christopher experience sensory play on a daily basis, not just during his play therapy sessions.

Christopher continued to engage in a lot of sensory play during the next phase of his therapy; he also began to explore some other play materials and started to engage in more projective play. Initially his projective play centred around sensory materials. From session 17 he began making things with the sensory materials rather than simply mixing random materials together. He regularly made playdough, delighting in the fact that he could chose his own colour and scent! Oobleck fascinated him, he loved the sensation of holding gloop ball in his hand and watching, and feeling, it turn into liquid. Slime made its way into the sessions, the therapist and Christopher worked together to get it to the consistency he enjoyed most. Stretchy slime, crunchy slime and foam slime were firm favourites, squeals of delight came from the room as the slime came together. The end product was also an incredible regulating and grounding tool for Christopher. As Christopher's play skills expanded so too did the play materials in the room. He was moving into projective play and towards role play so these play materials were returned to the play room. From session 20 on he was able to really engage and play with these. As he continued through his play therapy process he instinctively returned to sensory play whenever his body needed grounding. He continued to start and end the sessions with sensory play and if a play disruption occurred he found his way back to his favourite fidgets. Powerful abreactive play entered Christopher's therapy, he engaged in very deep process work in the later sessions in his therapy process.

When therapy ended, significant improvements were evident in each of the areas in which Christopher was initially experiencing difficulties. He had many positive relationships in his life, with family and friends, and was managing comfortably in school and at home. Final SDQ scores placed him in the normal/close to average in all categories. His overall impact score was 0, indicating no current trauma symptoms, and prosocial score was now 10, the most positive score on the scale.

The therapeutic powers of sensory play

This case study clearly illustrated Christopher's therapeutic use of sensory play in his psychotherapy sessions. This section highlights the actual mechanisms that effected change in Christopher, the activation of the four domains of the therapeutic powers of play (TPoP), incorporating all 20 of the core agents of change (Schaefer & Drewes, 2014). The TPoP will be italicised to easily identify them throughout this discussion.

In Christopher's very first play therapy session he had a strong reaction to the smell of the sand in the room. His physical response to the smell was intense, and was accompanied with verbalisations about the 'yucky smell'. He showed the therapist where he was at; through his limited vocalisation

Table 5.1 Therapeutic powers of play activated by Christopher through sensory play

Domain	Therapeutic powers of play
Facilitates communication	■ Self-expression ■ Access to the unconscious ■ Direct teaching ■ Indirect teaching
Fosters emotional wellness	■ Catharsis ■ Abreaction ■ Positive emotions ■ Counterconditioning of fears ■ Stress inoculation ■ Stress management
Enhances social relationships	■ Therapeutic relationship ■ Attachment ■ Social competence ■ Empathy
Increases personal strengths	■ Creative problem solving ■ Resiliency ■ Moral development ■ Accelerated psychological development ■ Self-regulation ■ Self-esteem

and his visceral reaction to the smell of the sand, he communicated his need for therapeutic sensory experiences (*self-expression*).

Christopher had little or no real play in his initial sessions. The sessions felt chaotic, frantic; Christopher was in and out of play, in and out of the playroom, in and out of connection with his parents and with the therapist. Sensory play was the gateway to Christopher's play. If a person is not regulated they cannot actually play (Prendiville, 2021). Clearly, age-appropriate state regulation was not established for Christopher. Sensory play worked to calm down Christopher's arousal system (*self-regulation*) and to stay in contact with the play materials, and with me (*therapeutic relationship*). In staying in contact with the materials he became fully engrossed and engaged. He adored the messy play, he experienced joy while engaging in it (*positive emotions*). There was a rapid increase in play, playfulness and mirth in the playroom. He began enjoying his individual play activities and the sensory play–based activities the therapist incorporated at the start and end of sessions with his parents (*positive emotions*). Fun and laughter now entered his relationship with his parents. He slowly began to be able to accept the comfort and regulation they offered him. Their relationship blossomed before the therapist's eyes. They experienced mutual joy and shared attention. The therapist witnessed the joyful lighting up of all of their eyes (*attachment*).

Sensory play was clearly very regulating for Christopher. The therapist recognised this and worked with his parents and teacher to help them to build in regular, repetitive sensory play experiences for Christopher. The increased use of sensory play in Christopher's everyday life proved very successful in helping him to soothe his nervous system and manage stress (*stress management*). Initially this play was adult led; in time Christopher's body began to recognise the sensory-based activities that regulated it, he automatically began going to those play-based activities when he needed them. He began to use sensory play at home and in school to help him to manage the ups and downs of everyday life (*self-regulation*).

Christopher's confidence and *self-esteem* grew as he played with the unstructured sensory play materials, he gained feelings of power and control. He set goals for himself and he reached them. Initially when the therapist met Christopher and his parents there had been a large emphasis in their interactions on controlling Christopher's behaviours and getting him to be a 'good boy'. During family sensory play times the therapist noticed that the focus on Christopher being 'good' was gone. Christopher was seen, accepted and valued by his parents for just being. The therapist noticed that Christopher began to experience strong feelings of power and control during his play therapy sessions (*self-esteem*). The therapists' use of esteem building responses while he engaged in sensory play also helped to bolster Christopher's *self-esteem*.

Sensory play provided Christopher with the ideal means to express his feelings and thoughts, and to help him to make sense of his experiences.

Christopher's real early life experiences were yucky, messy, disorganised and chaotic. His use of messy play in earlier sessions assisted him in gaining a sense of control over his world (*access to the unconscious*). He relished in playing around with the unknown and uncertainty of how things will work out. In later sessions, his repeated slime making provided him with further opportunities to explore these personally relevant themes. He managed big feelings of disappointment, frustration and anger, which arose during the play. He began to accept help, to be able to tolerate the uncertainty in some of his play, to work through his big feelings and to understand and gain control of them.

Christopher's engagement in sensory play expanded his understanding of himself and the world around him. It provided him with opportunities to practise and develop a multitude of skills. The initial sensory play–based sessions with Christopher were very interactive in nature. The therapist's aim was to enrich his play by engaging and connecting with him. Joint attention and mutual joy (*positive emotions*) enabled the facilitation of a two-way interaction through play. Christopher's engagement in sensory play fostered development across all psychological domains; it also improved his play skills and enabled him to move into projective and role play. This development in his play skills then allowed him to access the developmental benefits associated with the more cognitive forms of play (*accelerated psychological development*).

Pretend play is often associated with *creative problem solving* (Russ & Wallace, 2014). Christopher's engagement in sensory play also facilitated his development of problem solving skills. He practised divergent thinking, engaged with real-life challenges when figuring out what to add in when his playdough was too sticky, or too dry, and of course when mastering his slime-making techniques. As Christopher's play progressed, he moved further into role play and his *creative problem solving* abilities became even more apparent.

Blundon Nash (2014, p. 187) states that '[d]evelopmentally, one of the earliest forms of play in which children engage that promotes acquisition of social skills is rough and tumble play'. The therapist took on the role of the regulated other during rough and tumble play, and she supported his parents to do the same. This enabled Christopher to remain cheerful, playful and non-aggressive while engaging in rough and tumble play in the therapy room, and at home, thus ensuring it had a positive impact on his *social competence*. Christopher began to show his developing *social competence* in the therapy room, at home and at school. He started dividing out his messy play creations between himself and the therapist in the playroom, he began sharing with other children in school, and engaging in turn-taking games at home with his parents. Christopher's ability to pay attention to another, to plan and work together was clear in his social interactions.

Gaskill (2014) explores the positive impact of repetitive sensory-motor play and nurturing physical play on the development of *empathy*. Christopher's regular engagement in sensory-motor play, physical play and nurturing interactions with his parents and his therapist appears to have resulted in affective empathic learning and an overall increase in his *empathy*. This became very evident during his later role play and when his developing *empathy* began to show in his relationships with his peers and the adults in his life.

Sensory play worked to calm Christopher's arousal system, which allowed him to stay in contact with the play materials and with others. The regular use of sensory play in his home enabled him to interact more fully with his parents and to strengthen his relationship with them. The use of non-directive commentary also supported the strengthening of these significant relationships. Both Kohlberg and Piaget identified the need for interaction and relationship to support the development of morality (Packman, 2014, p. 247). When Christopher began his therapy journey he became angry easily, he regularly lashed out at others: hitting, kicking and biting them. He showed no remorse or understanding of how his actions impacted on those around him. His actions were generally met with anger and discipline. In the therapy room Christopher's messy play, his messy explosions, were met with acceptance and reflection. His parents learnt to meet his play with acceptance and reflection too; they began to use the same principles when responding to his challenging behaviours. Safety limits were set when necessary, Christopher accepted these and began to demonstrate a genuine awareness of the need for limits and the impact of his actions on others. He developed an ability to accept and express empathy and understanding *(moral development)*.

In abreactive play children re-enact and relive stressful and traumatic experiences, often in symbolic form, and thus gain a sense of power and control of them (Prendiville, 2014a). Christopher's hide and find games with the therapist in the playroom were highly charged and extremely significant. The addition of rhythmic clapping by the therapist as she searched for Christopher in various tiny spaces added to the sensory experience of the game. Her genuine delight each time she found Christopher was mutual and extremely reparative for Christopher. The activation of Christopher's PLAY system (Panksepp, 1998) enabled Christopher to engage with the difficult emotions associated with his early life abandonment *(abreaction)*.

Catharsis allows for the release and completion of previously restrained or interrupted affective release via emotional expression or activity (Drewes & Schaefer, 2014). While engaging in sensory play Christopher physically expressed and released tensions in a safe and progressive way *(catharsis)*. Week after week his use of sensory play in the therapy room enabled him to purge his emotional distress and experience relief and psychological calm. His daily sensory play experiences at home and in school allowed him to experience *catharsis* on a regular and repetitive basis.

Christopher's sensory play experiences included lots of uncertainty, it afforded him many opportunities to take risks, to problem solve, to create meaning, to manage uncertainty and to develop coping skills within the safety of play. As the therapy progressed Christopher demonstrated a growing sense of confidence, competence, connection and control in his play. These skills soon began to transfer over into his relationships and everyday interactions enabling him to deal successfully with adjustments, stressors and novel situations (*resiliency*).

Sensory play was also the platform that enabled the therapist to make use of some of the other TPoP. Sensory play worked to calm Christopher's arousal system, establish safety and play and foster a strong *therapeutic relationship*, enabling activation of many of the TPoP. After repeated sensory play experiences the therapist was able to use *direct teaching* and *indirect teaching* through the use of puppets, stories and role play with Christopher. The therapist utilised playful *stress inoculation* strategies to prepare Christopher for potentially stressful events and more directive play techniques to support his *counterconditioning of fears*. Through sensory play Christopher developed his ability to engage in rich role play; in the later stages of Christopher's play therapy his role play was *abreactive*. These would not have been possible in the early stages of Christopher's therapy when his imaginative play skills were less developed. In examining Christopher's entire psychotherapy process it is evident that Christopher's regulation, through sensory play, opened up the pathway for all of the other TPoP to activate. Sensory play was key in Christopher's psychotherapy journey; for him it was certainly a powerful enzyme that aided his digestion of unresolved material and overwhelming emotions. Through sensory play he found himself, his joy, his happiest, healthiest way of being.

Conclusion

This chapter has brought together evidence from the literature, established therapies and clinical practice to bring the therapeutic powers of sensory play to life. In linking theory with practice-based knowledge, the key specific change agents in sensory play were identified and the incredible power of sensory play to act as a gateway to illuminate all of the TPoP. The articulation of a strong theoretical and clinical rationale for the integration of sensory play in psychotherapy and play therapy aims to strengthen and inform the clinician's practice and their understanding of the application of the therapeutic powers of play.

References

Beckerleg, T. (2009). *Fun with messy play: Ideas and activities for children with special needs.* London: Jessica Kingsley.

Blundon Nash, J. (2014). Social competence. In C. E. Schaefer & A. A. Drewes (Eds.) *The therapeutic powers of play: 20 core agents of change* (2nd ed., pp. 185–195). Hoboken, NJ: Wiley.

Booth, P. B., & Jernberg, A. M. (2010). *Theraplay: Helping parents and children build better relationships through attachment-based play* (3rd ed.). San Francisco, CA: John Wiley.

Brody, V. A. (1978, November). Developmental play: A relationship-focused program for children. In *Child Welfare Journal of Policy, Practice, and Program, 57*(9), 591–599.

Brody, V. A. (1993). *The dialogue of touch: Developmental play therapy.* Treasure Island, FL: Developmental Play Training Associates.

Bruce, T. (2011). *Learning through play for babies, toddlers and young children* (2nd ed.). London: Hodder Education.

Cozolino, L. (2010). *The neuroscience of psychotherapy: Healing the social brain.* New York: W. W. Norton.

Drewes, A., & Schaefer, C. E. (2014). Catharsis. In C. E. Schaefer & A. A. Drewes (Eds.), *The therapeutic powers of play: 20 core agents of change* (2nd ed., pp. 71–83). Hoboken, NJ: Wiley.

Fearn, M. (2014). Working therapeutically with groups in the outdoors: A natural space for healing. In E. Prendiville & J. Howard (Eds.), *Play therapy today: Contemporary practice for individuals, groups and carers* (pp. 7–28). London: Routledge.

Gascoyne, S. (2011). *Sensory play: Play in the EYFS.* London: MA Education Ltd.

Gaskill, R. (2014). Empathy. In C. E. Schaefer & A. A. Drewes (Eds.), *The therapeutic powers of play: 20 core agents of change* (2nd ed., pp. 195–207). Hoboken, NJ: Wiley.

Godwin Emmons, P., & McKendry Anderson, L. (2005). *Understanding sensory dysfunction: Learning, development and sensory dysfunction in autism spectrum disorders, ADHD, learning disabilities and bipolar disorder.* London: Jessica Kingsley Publishers.

Goodman, R. (1997). The strengths and difficulties questionnaire: A research note. *Journal of Child Psychology and Psychiatry, 38*, 581–586.

Harvey, S. A. (1994). Dynamic play therapy: Expressive play interventions with families. In K. O'Connor & C. E. Schaefer (Eds.). *Handbook of play therapy, advances and innovations* (vol. 2, pp. 85–110). Hoboken, NJ: Wiley.

Harvey, S. A. (2008). Dynamic play with very young children. In C. E. Schaefer, S. Kelly-Zion, J. McCormick, and A. Ohnogi (Eds.), *Play therapy for very young children.* (pp. 3–23). Livingston, NJ: Aronson.

Jennings, S. (1999). *Introduction to developmental play therapy.* London: Jessica Kingsley.

Jennings, S. (2011). *Healthy attachments and neuro-dramatic-play.* London: Jessica Kingsley.

Landreth, G. (2012). *Play therapy: The art of the relationship.* (3rd ed.). New York: Routledge.

Nelson, J. (2008). Laugh and the world laughs with you: An attachment perspective on the meaning of laughter in psychotherapy. *Clinical Social Work Journal, 36*(1), 41–49.

Packman, J. (2014). Moral development. In C. E. Schaefer & A. A. Drewes (Eds.), *The therapeutic powers of play: 20 core agents of change* (2nd ed., pp. 243–254). Hoboken, NJ: Wiley.

Panksepp, J. (1998). *Affective neuroscience: The foundations of human and animal emotions*. New York, NY: Oxford University Press.

Perry, B. D. (2006). Applying principles of neurodevelopment to clinical work with maltreated and traumatized children. In N. B. Webb (Ed.), *Working with traumatized youth in child welfare* (pp. 27–52). New York: Guilford Press.

Prendiville, E. (2014b). The therapeutic touchstone. In E. Prendiville & J. Howard (Eds.), *Creative psychotherapy: Applying the principles of neurobiology to play and expressive arts-based practice* (pp. 7–28). Oxon: Routledge.

Prendiville, E. (2014a). Abreaction. In C. E. Schaefer & A. A. Drewes (Eds.) *The therapeutic powers of play: 20 core agents of change* (2nd ed., pp. 83–103). Hoboken, NJ: Wiley.

Prendiville, S. (2014). Accelerated psychological development. In C. E. Schaefer & A. A. Drewes (Eds.), *The therapeutic powers of play: 20 core agents of change* (2nd ed., pp. 255–268). Hoboken, NJ: Wiley.

Prendiville, S. (2021). Sensory play therapy. In H. G. Kaduson & C. E. Schaefer (Eds.), *Play therapy with children: Modalities for change* (pp. 157–176). American Psychological Association.

Prendiville, S., & Fearn, M. (2017). Coming alive: Finding joy through sensory play. In E. Prendiville & J. Howard (Eds.), *Creative psychotherapy: Applying the principles of neurobiology to play and expressive arts-based practice* (pp. 121–137). Oxon: Routledge.

Russ, S. W., & Wallace, C. E. (2014). *Creative problem solving*. In C. E. Schaefer & A. A. Drewes (Eds.), *The therapeutic powers of play: 20 core agents of change* (2nd ed., pp. 213–225). Hoboken, NJ: Wiley.

Schaefer, C. E., & Drewes, A. A. (Eds.) (2014). *The therapeutic powers of play: 20 core agents of change* (2nd ed.) Hoboken, NJ: Wiley.

Schore, A. N. (2005). Attachment, affect and the developing right brain: Linking developmental neuroscience to pediatrics. *Pediatric Review*, 26, 2014–2017.

Schore, J., & Schore, A. (2008). Modern attachment theory: The central role of affect regulation in development and treatment. *Clinical Social Work Journal*, 36, 9–20.

Stagnitti, K. (1998). *Learn to play. A program to develop a child's imaginative play skills*. Melbourne: Co-ordinates Publications.

Stagnitti, K. (2009). Play intervention: The learn to play program. In K. Stagnitti & R. Cooper (Eds.), *Play as therapy* (pp. 87–101). London, England: Kingsley.

Usher, W. (2010). *Sensory play resource book*. London: Kids.

Yasenik, L., & Gardner, K. (2012). *Play therapy dimensions model: A decision making guide for integrative play therapists*. Philadelphia, PA: Jessica Kingsley Publications.

Chapter 6

It's a small world: Projective play

Kate L. Renshaw and Judi A. Parson

Introduction

Projective play is critical for the discovery of the self. Play permits self-discovery within safe and developmentally adaptable parameters. Winnicott (1971, p. 54) described that 'it is in playing and only in playing that the individual child or adult is able to be creative and to use the whole personality, and it is only in being creative that the individual discovers the self'. Jennings (2011) details the Embodiment-Projection-Role (EPR) sequence from birth to seven years of age and beyond, with a focus period on projective play occurring between 13 months and three years of age. Cattanach (2003, p. 33) states that 'projective play happens when the child discovers the world outside themselves through toys, dolls and other play objects'. In normative play development, projective play aligns with several phases of the eight psychosocial stages in Erikson's (1963) human development theory: namely autonomy vs. shame and doubt, initiative vs. guilt and industry vs. inferiority (see Table 6.1). Erikson's stages each have an approximate age range and a key word for each stage; for the projective phase, *will, purpose* and *competence* are developmentally significant (Kinnick & Wells, 2014).

Erikson's stages of psychosocial development and Jennings' (1999) EPR will be integrated with the Therapeutic Powers of Play (TPoP) (Schaefer & Drewes, 2014) to set the scene for the case study. This chapter aims to (1) define small world play, (2) provide an historical overview of the use of small world play, (3) explore the play therapy theoretical foundations of small world play, (4) outline the developmental benefits of projective play and (5) extrapolate the therapeutic value of projective play and small world play for children attending play therapy.

Definition of projective play

Projective play is a style of play which can be identified by using dolls and other toys to facilitate expression of feelings (American Psychological Association, 2020a). Specifically, 'in psychoanalytic and psychodynamic

Table 6.1 Childhood psychosocial stages

Age	Keyword	Stage
Birth to 1.5 years	HOPE	Trust vs. Mistrust
1.5–3 years	WILL	Autonomy vs. Shame and doubt
3–6 years	PURPOSE	Initiative vs. Guilt
6–13 years	COMPETENCE	Industry vs. Inferiority
13–18 years	FIDELITY	Identify vs. Role confusion

theories, the process by which one attributes one's own individual positive or negative characteristics, affects, and impulses to another person or group' (APA Dictionary of Psychology, 2020b). Projecting parts of the self externally onto objects or expressive arts materials can provide a safe psychological distance in order to 'draw from within' to externalise internal thoughts and feelings (Malchiodi, 2007, p. 4). Following a review of the play therapy literature, scant publications were found on projective play. The main scholars on projective play within play therapy literature are Sue Jennings (1999, 2011, 2014) and Ann Cattanach (2003). Projective play is defined by Jennings (2014) as 'play beyond the body' (p. 85). This type of play enables children to explore, respond and connect with the world outside of themselves. *Projective* play often appears as more controlled and ordered in style and builds on the sensory (e.g. mess-making) and emotional exploration on the previous phase of play *embodiment* (Jennings, 2014). Projection can be described as building, making, creating and narrating. Examples of projective play resources include construction toys and materials, dolls house, miniature figurines, unstructured objects for scene setting, building and creating, a range of art/craft materials, playdough and clay with sculpting tools and sand and water play resources (Cattanach, 2003, Jennings, 1999, 2014). Projective play is broad and encompasses many variants of projection and projective materials. However, for the scope of this chapter, we will focus in on small world play as a sub-type of projective play.

Definition of small world play

Small world play is a common term used in early years education practice and publications. Normative small world play experience for children in early education settings use objects, toys and play scenes to invite children to explore real-life experiences or create their own stories. Small world play in play therapy is differentiated from normative small world play in educative settings by taking place within a therapeutic environment, relationship and with careful choice of resources by the therapist.

Small world resources in play therapy include playdough and clay, dollhouse with furniture and figures, other buildings (such as police station, castle, hospital, pirate ship, fire station, etc.), vehicles, play mats, sand tray, water tray, range of miniature figurines and a range of miniaturised unstructured objects, including natural materials (see additional resources for more ideas). There is sparse literature in play therapy on small world play.

An historical overview of small world play

Children's play and their toys have long been of interest to archaeologists around the world. Toys are on the shortlist of artefacts recovered from ancient human civilisations (Sommer & Sommer, 2017). Miniaturised wheeled horses and dolls date back to Ancient Greece some 2,500 years ago (Sommer 2017). There is evidence to suggest that small world play may have existed for 4,000 years. A doll buried with miniature-sized kitchenware found in Italy may indicate that small world and projective play could be as old as the most ancient civilisations (Williams, 2012). 'Children at play everywhere and across time take advantage of the opportunities that toys afford them' (Sommer & Sommer, 2017, p. 353).

In 1730, toy soldiers were the first miniatures to be manufactured commercially (Garson, 2013). Miniature toys grew in popularity, and by the Victorian era small dolls and clockwork toys such as miniature trains accompanied the toy soldiers (Coşkunsu, 2015). H. G. Wells' pivotal text *Floor Games*, first published in 1911, detailed the toys and play of his own children (Wells, 1911). He defined four main categories of miniature toys: (1) soldiers, (2) bricks, (3) boards and planks and (4) clockwork railway rolling stock and rails (Turner, 2004).

From the play and stories of children and families as depicted in *Floor Games,* the first-known therapeutic application of projective small world play into child therapy occurred (Turner, 2004). Margaret Lowenfeld, inspired by the writings of H. G. Wells, started to incorporate similar small world toys into her clinical work (Hutton, 2004; Turner, 2004). Combining small world toys and her clinical experience of how child clients utilised these play materials, Lowenfeld created the World Technique. Lowenfeld advised five main categories of miniature toys: (1) living creatures, (2) fantasy and folklore, (3) scenery, (4) transport and (5) equipment (Hutton, 2004). She also advised having a miscellaneous category such as natural found objects (Hutton, 2004). These categories of small world toys may then be used within the various spheres of play (Erikson, 1972, 1977).

Erikson (1972) observed and theorised there to be three spheres of play: (1) autosphere, (2) microsphere and (3) macrosphere. The microsphere is the sphere that aligns with small world play; in the microsphere 'the child plays in a miniature toy world, usually using miniature replicas or substitutes for real objects' (Chazan, 2002, p. 35). The microsphere affords the greatest freedom of all three spheres as exploration occurs within the miniaturised world of small world play (Chazan, 2002). A modern-day example of projective/small world toys being acknowledged for their importance came in 2008. The stick was officially inducted into the toy hall of fame as potentially the oldest toy in the world (National Museum of Play, n.d.). Sticks may be used in all three spheres of play, for example a stick could extend a finger or limb as part of their body, it could be used as a fence in a play scene or used as a wand to project a magic spell.

Theoretical rationale for small world play

When incorporating projective small world play into their play therapy rooms, the authors consciously base their clinical reasoning on integrative theoretical foundations. Aspects of practice that are affected by theoretical foundations include the following: choice of toys and expressive materials, the style of the therapeutic relationship and tracking the themes of the play therapy and the therapeutic process. For the authors, the use of small world play within play therapy is based on five integrated theoretical foundations: (1) humanistic play therapy, (2) TPoP, (3) Eriksonian psychosocial developmental stages, (4) neuro-dramatic play (NDP) and (5) EPR.

Humanistic approaches in psychotherapy, including humanistic play therapy 'view the relationship between the child and the therapist as the vehicle for dynamic growth and healing' (Bratton & Ray, 2002, p. 370). Humanistic play therapy skills can be attributed to Carl Rogers (1957), Clark Moustakas (1959), Virginia Axline (1964; 1969), Donald Winnicott (1965; 1971) and Mary Ainsworth (van Rosmalen, van der Horst & van der Veer, 2016). These are summarised in Table 6.2, attributing the skill to the scholar.

The humanistic play therapy skills are important as a collective stance in order to enter the world of the child to facilitate therapeutic play within a secure and safe relationship and environment. The following schemata (Figure 6.1) represents the integration of humanistic play therapy skills which promote the creation of optimal conditions for children to engage in projective small world play.

Table 6.2 Attribution of humanistic play therapy skills

Scholar	Humanistic skill
Carl Rogers	Empathy, unconditional positive regard (UPR) and congruence
Clark Moustakas and Virginia Axline	Limitations with UPR and empathy
Virginia Axline	Tracking, structuring, limits and routines
Donald Winnicott	Being, doing, joining and holding
Mary Ainsworth	Attunement

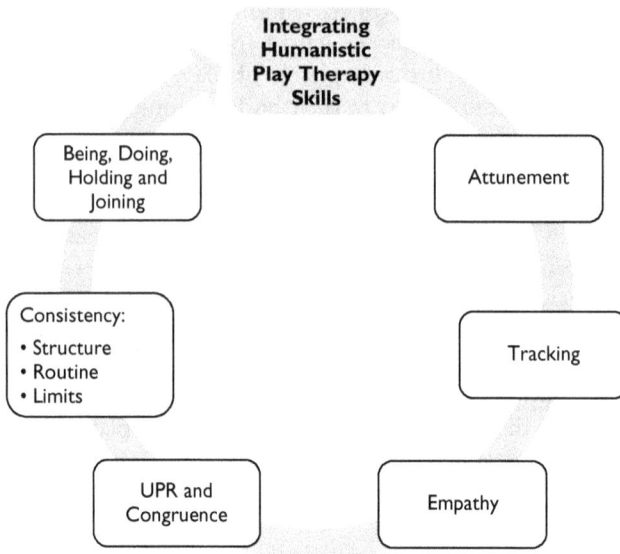

Figure 6.1 Integrating humanistic play therapy skills.

The schemata outlining the optimal conditions for play therapy sets the scene to introduce an extended theoretical framework for understanding how play facilitates change. These change agents are known as the TPoP and are described by Schaefer & Drewes (2014) as 'the essence, the "heart and soul" of play therapy' (p. 4). The authors propose that humanistic play therapy skills (Figure 6.1) and the TPoP (see Figure 1.1) complement each other to form the art and science of play therapy.

Turning the clock back to Erikson's world view helps to situate how his psychosocial stages (as outlined in Table 6.1) supports contemporary play therapists to hypothesise, assess, track therapeutic progress and define play themes (Ryan & Edge, 2012). As such, Eriksonian psychosocial stages are an essential component incorporated into this integrative theoretical rationale for planning, implementing and understanding projective small world play.

Projective play and small world play have been largely conceptualised in the writing of Sue Jennings (1999). Jennings (2014) states that there is a theoretical bridge between drama therapy and play therapy and describes these two developmental therapeutic approaches as akin to a DNA helix. NDP and EPR have strengthened the theoretical foundations of play therapy in relation to the developmental and biological basis for play and health. Based on neuroscience and attachment knowledge, NDP is primarily focussed on child and play development commencing between three months gestation until six months of age (Jennings, 2014). Whereas, EPR begins from birth and merges with NDP throughout the development of the child and their sequential play development (Jennings, 2014). Jennings (2014) states that NDP and EPR are both vital for normative child development and well-being. They can also be restorative for children engaged in play therapy and can support the therapist's clinical reasoning; 'rather like the chains of DNA, NDP and EPR create curls and swirls of how we think about the creative play process and how we apply it' (Jennings, 2014, p. 81).

Developmental benefits of projective play

There are numerous neuro-bio-psycho-social benefits to children when engaging in projective and small world play. Most children, unless developing atypically, engage in play intuitively. Play supports the growth and development of children's brains from the bottom up. Play also supports bodily development through both fine motor and gross motor engagement in playful experiences. From the first playful parenting moments through to social engagement with peers, children develop socially and emotionally because of relational play experiences. Projective play allows children to externalise internal thoughts and feelings onto toys and creative materials outside the body. This facilitates safe self-expression and self-exploration, which may be accessed throughout childhood. From a developmental perspective, small world play is integrated as part of the EPR sequence and is significant between three and ten years of age. Projective small world play can be accessed and paced by the child. However, Stagnitti (2009) states that play is an ability and as such not all children can self-initiate play. While pretend play skills develop first through a combination of embodiment play and projective play, e.g. body scripts where a child feeds themselves and a teddy bear (Stagnitti, 1998). As pretend play skills develop, the incorporation of small world play resources, including unstructured objects, such as a stick, a piece of fabric and a cardboard shoebox, may allow children to extend their play narratives (Stagnitti, 1998). Object substitution, whereby random objects can be used in play by children to become whatever the child wishes, e.g. a cardboard shoe box becomes a car for the teddy, has been found to be a threshold concept for children as they hone their pretend play skills (Stagnitti, 1998). Once a child unlocks their potential for pretending that an object can be anything, then their imaginative play skills develop rapidly. With the ability to play imaginatively 'toys and objects assist the child in externalisation and help the child to separate from a problem and expand their perspectives' (Cattanach, 2003, p. 33). Most importantly, imaginative, pretend play skills are transformative, allowing a shift into the next phase of the EPR sequence, i.e. from projective play to role play.

The developmental benefits of projective small world play (Jennings, 1999; 2011) can be aligned with Erikson's (1957) psychosocial stages. As highlighted in Table 6.1, three of Erikson's psychosocial stages can be mapped in relation to projective small world play and associated developmental benefits and resources. Firstly, young children (1.5–3 years) are developing their sense of *autonomy*, this supports them to begin to explore beyond their own body and thus marks the commencement of projective play. Projective play within co-regulated relationships supports emotional and bodily exploration and expression as children develop their sense of autonomy. Resources that scaffold children into autonomous play experiences include large-sized building blocks and toys as well as unstructured objects. Secondly, children (three to six years) move onto developing their sense of *initiative*; this stage sees a deepening exploration of personal interests, facilitated by their increasing projective play skills. Child development is enriched through the exploration of the child's interests, things going well and being enjoyable, things going not so well and learning to cope with setbacks, solving problems, and being innovative and experimental. Resources that support children to explore their developing sense of initiative include small toys, building blocks, small cars, first puzzles and a diverse range of unstructured objects. Thirdly, in middle childhood (6–11 years) children are developing their sense of *industry*. Projective small world play can be an entry point for children to explore their growing sense of industry through play. They may choose play or narrative scenarios to protectively explore their own thoughts and feelings as well as trialling and potentially finding solutions to problems. There may be setbacks as children navigate these experiences, but with increasing industry comes increased feelings of pride and enjoyment. Children's growing sense of industry supports them to independently choose play materials that they find engaging and enjoyable. Miniature figurines, dolls houses, sand and water trays may facilitate industrious expression. It is important to note that access to more sophisticated arts and craft materials enhances independence and choice when engaging in projective play.

Case study

Amber, an eight-year-old girl, was referred to play therapy because of anxiety related to witnessing a serious scene of family violence, which required the hospitalisation and rehabilitation of her mother. Amber attended 16 sessions of individual humanistic play therapy before transitioning into filial therapy with her mother; however, this case example focusses only on the individual play therapy component. All clinical sessions took place in a community-based setting attached to a school. The case study is structured sequentially as clusters from early, middle and final sessions. Exemplars are used to illustrate the therapeutic use of projective and small world play as well as the activation of the four domains of the TPoP which incorporates 19 of the 20 core agents of change throughout Amber's play therapy (see Table 6.3) (Schaefer & Drewes, 2014). The TPoP will be italicised to easily identify them throughout this case presentation.

Table 6.3 Therapeutic powers of play activated by Amber through projective play

Domain	Therapeutic powers of play
Facilitates communication	■ Self-expression ■ Access to the unconscious ■ Indirect teaching ■ Direct teaching
Increases personal strengths	■ Self-esteem ■ Creative problem solving ■ Resiliency ■ Accelerated psychological development ■ Moral development ■ Self-regulation
Fosters emotional wellness	■ Catharsis ■ Counterconditioning fears ■ Abreaction ■ Positive emotions ■ Stress inoculation ■ Stress management
Enhances social relationships	■ Empathy ■ Attachment ■ Therapeutic relationship

Early sessions

The *therapeutic relationship* with Amber started from the first time that she walked into the playroom and throughout the course of the therapeutic intervention. The *therapeutic relationship* was initiated through relational style *attachment* play. For example, she loved to play catch with the Balzac ball, a soft but waterproof fabric covering a balloon, she delighted in throwing it back and forth – connecting through a safe distance but in a fun way. Due to Amber's experience of family violence, she needed to spend the early phase of therapy establishing a trusting relationship with the therapist. Amber explored her developing sense of safety in the relationship (sense of *attachment*) through emulating some of the early projective play of younger children, such as vocal hide-and-seek, rhythmic musical instrument follow the leader and a generalised sense of felt security from an attuned sensitive adult (the play therapist).

As Amber's therapeutic process progressed, she shifted into projective and small world play, the *therapeutic relationship* remained stable and

Amber was able to engage and deepen her projective play in the therapeutic presence of the therapist, so much so she would seek and invite the therapist in as a co-player. For example, Amber would use symbols and play out scenes of danger (miniature figurines of snakes and spiders) while at the same time Amber directed the therapist to play out protective dynamics (miniature figurines of mother and baby) to elaborate relational safety within a complex small world narrative sequence. Amber seemed to be searching for a safe protective space from danger. As play therapy progressed, themes of trust in others facilitated a sense of trust in self developing (*self-esteem*).

Mid-sessions

During the mid-session phase of play therapy, a trusting *therapeutic relationship* was strengthening. Amber increased in confidence to engage in a range of projective play that facilitated many moments to experience, embody and internalise *positive emotions*. She found joy in relational moments while co-creating art, for example Amber would state 'you draw the flower and I'll draw the tree' or during game play, for example 'let's play Jenga®' and watching and delighting in the tensions between stability and instability. From this mid-stage of therapy, these joyful moments occurred with increasing frequency throughout the therapeutic intervention.

Towards the end of the mid-session phase of play therapy, Amber engaged with the Playmobil® Take Along Pirate Island with additional Playmobil® figurines to ensure a balanced range of projective resources. This resource included miniature pirate figures and magical fairy figures and other props such as boats, trees, treasure chests and animals such as a unicorn, swan and peacock, etc. During a significant session Amber set up the small world scene and then played out the story of a little fairy girl and her fairy mother (see Figure 6.2). The fairy mother played happily with her fairy daughter, but, one day, pirates came. The fairy mother was frightened and hid the fairy daughter away in a large treasure chest. The pirates attacked the fairy mother repeatedly and, all the while, the fairy girl hid safely in the chest, but she saw everything that happened to the fairy mother. This small world play scene formed the basis of a very intense play therapy session for Amber. She felt able to use the small world play materials to express and attempt to make sense of the brutal attack on the fairy mother. During the play scene and on further reflection after the therapy session the therapist identified that Amber had been able to *access her unconscious* and *self-express* her own experience of being shut away in a cupboard by her mother to be protected from a family violence scenario that left her mother fighting for her life in a hospital.

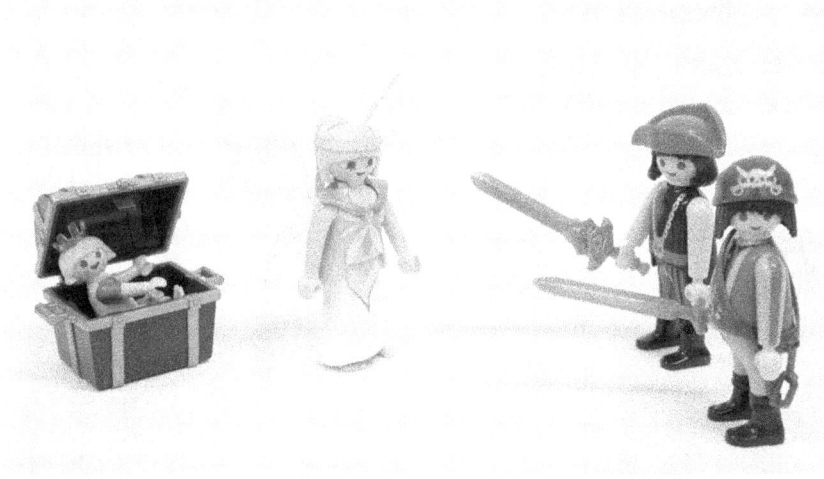

Figure 6.2 Playmobil® Pirate Island and fairy figurines.

The pirate island play scene allowed Amber to foster her emotional wellness through *abreactive* play and *cathartic expression*. By using small world play Amber was able to re-create the scene of family violence in miniaturised scale and with the safe distance that play affords. Amber re-played the scene of the day of the family violence that led to her mother's hospitalisation. She was able to release difficult feelings through this play process which resulted in *cathartic* release. The scale of the miniaturised play scene allowed Amber to 'be in charge' of this frightening story while remaining at a safe psychological distance. The therapist's use of humanistic skills, such as tracking and empathically reflecting, helped to reanimate Amber's narrative of the story of the fairy daughter, fairy mother and the pirates. The pirate island play had also activated Amber's ability to explore and further develop her social conscience and thus *moral development*. Through this play scenario, Amber explored what it means for humans to be good and/or bad, kind and/or unkind.

During the final sessions of play therapy, Amber remembered the pirate ship play and decided to use the projective art materials to create a drawn scene of the pirate ship. She created the scene using sophisticated art materials (oil pastels and graphite pencils). The artwork she created was developmentally very sophisticated compared to her previous art making and was well above the typical drawing development indicators for her age. This self-motivated projective drawing creation highlighted Amber's *accelerated psychological development* as part of her therapeutic process.

Final sessions

Towards the end of individual play therapy sessions, Amber had an accident where she was required to go to the accident and emergency unit at a local hospital. Amber had stood on a rusted nail that was sticking out of the fence she was trying to climb over. The nail was removed but bled profusely at the farm. Once cleaned and bandaged she was advised to have a tetanus vaccination, however she became so dysregulated that she refused to have the injection. An appointment was rescheduled to give Amber time to prepare for the injection. Amber's mother contacted the play therapist and sought additional support. The therapist suggested a one-off directive session with both Amber and her mother to scaffold and support Amber ahead of the scheduled injection. The therapist prepared Amber for this more directive session, as a one-off purposive format, in contrast to the usual individual humanistic play therapy sessions. Amber was relieved that the play therapist was aware of the recent difficult experience of the vaccination injection and said that 'I really hope Mum can help me when I have to have the real needle'.

At the start of this directive session, the therapist invited Amber to choose a calico doll, which come in a range of skin colour tones (see Figure 6.3), and to decorate the doll and give the doll a name. Amber created her doll and called it Ella. The therapist then used Ella to teach Amber and her mother how to use the 'magic glove' technique (Kuttner, 2012), a type of hypnosis to potentially reduce felt pain in medical procedures (see recommended resources section). They also practised using a 'buzzy', which combines a cold

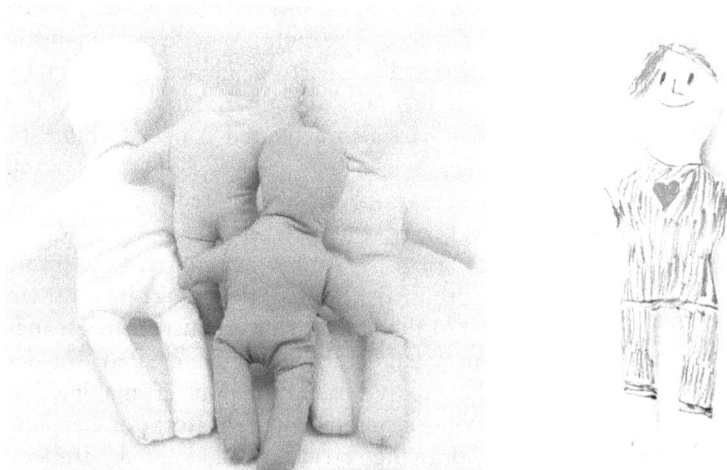

Figure 6.3 Calico dolls showing colour variations and Ella the calico doll.

pack with a vibrating bee that is placed between the site of the injection and the brain, interrupting pain signals (see additional resources section). Procedural medical play, using projective play resources, enabled Amber to prepare in a step-by-step way for her upcoming injection. This segment of the play session was focussed on *direct and indirect teaching* by the therapist. After both supportive medical methods were practised with Amber, she then had the opportunity to teach Ella about these procedures too. In this segment of the play session Amber was able to experience *stress inoculation* when she used Ella as a pretend patient to teach Ella about injections through projective play. The projective play with Ella and the medical kit (role-play materials) allowed Amber to explore and mange her stresses (*stress management*) about the repeated injection she was being preparing for. This play session also supported Amber in *counterconditioning fear* as well as providing *stress inoculation* for future medical procedures.

Amber was then invited by the therapist to use the playroom in a non-directive manner. Amber chose to take Ella (see Figure 6.3) on an exploratory journey around the playroom where she introduced Ella to her favourite toys.

Amber decided to make Ella some more friends out of the arts and craft materials. She used unstructured objects to create other characters; the complexity of object substitution, creativity and strong narrative displayed *accelerated psychological development*. Amber made two new friends for Ella, called Tom and Sarah. Tom (see Figure 6.4) was created by sticking feathers, sticks and facial features to a play phone in the playroom and Sarah (see Figure 6.4) was created by sticking a pre-made half face mask, a peg and pipe cleaners to a piece of cardboard that had been cut to shape using crinkle-cut craft scissors.

Amber knew the rule in the playroom that the toys were for staying in the playroom so that they could be available in subsequent session. However, she had her heart set on taking Tom home with Ella and Sarah. This projective play sequence enabled Amber to explore her sense of *self-regulation* when faced with her range of emotions around the rules of the playroom. She was also able to *creatively problem solve*, which saw her take apart and reassemble Tom onto a new base (a piece of cardboard cut to the size of the phone). Finally, this supported Amber to build *resilience* through the process of navigating these challenging and emotionally difficult moments.

As this session drew to an end, Amber was able to show her increased sense of *empathy* to others through her playful relationship with Ella. It is important to acknowledge that this could only be achieved following a prolonged *therapeutic relationship* over 16 sessions. It is interesting to note that a parallel process was unfolding when previously the therapist modelling attunement and empathy to Amber, which in turn facilitated opportunities for Amber to demonstrate similar sensitive caring messages to

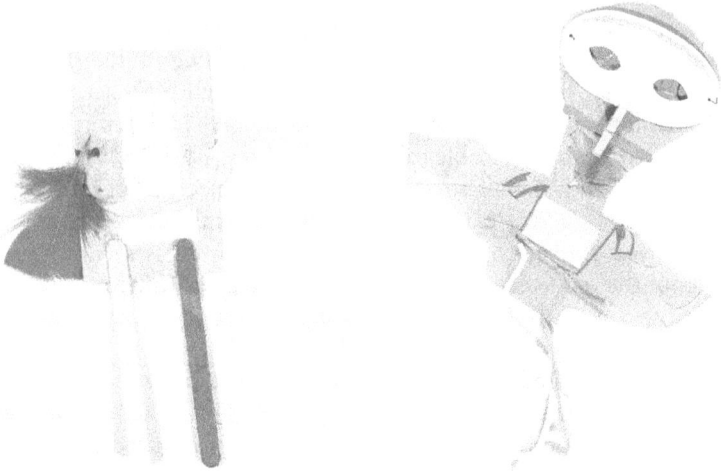

Figure 6.4 Tom and Sarah.

Ella. With her the projective toy creations, Amber was able to express *empathy* towards Ella when she was practising giving Ella an injection. Amber extended this *empathic response* when she was able to consider not only her own but other children's and even her own pet cat's experience of needling procedures.

Conclusion

Projective play, especially small world play is recognised and valued in play therapy. This type of play can be tailored to the individual through the provision of developmentally sensitive play and creative resources. Understanding the historical development of projective play has mapped how this type of play has been integrated into play therapy. Articulating a strong theoretical rationale for the importance of small world play in play therapy strengthens and informs practice. Play practitioners may wish to advocate for projective, small world play in a variety of settings, including community-based, schools and in the home with the parents and families. The case example of Amber has brought to life how projective play, especially small world play harmonises with the TPoP to provide the rich therapeutic conditions for healing and growth within humanistic play therapy. Further research and publications into projective and small world play are recommended to increase literature and resources for practitioners.

Additional resources

- Miniature figures (Homeyer & Sweeney, 2017, p. 25–37).
- Practical play therapy: Projection (Jennings, 1999, p. 101–118).
- Applying an embodiment-projection-role framework in group work with children (Jennings, 2014, p. 81–96).
- Appendix 2 – embodiment-projection-role (0–7 years) (Jennings, 2011, p. 247–254).
- The magic glove – hypnotic pain management for children https://www.youtube.com/watch?v=cyApK8Z_SQQ.
- Buzzy-pain relief https://buzzyhelps.com/.

References

American Psychological Association (2020a). *APA Dictionary of Psychology*. Retrieved from https://dictionary.apa.org/projective-play.

American Psychological Association (2020b). *APA Dictionary of Psychology*. Retrieved from https://dictionary.apa.org/projection.

Axline, V. M. (1964). *Dibs: In search of self.* New York: Ballantine Books.

Axline, V. M. (1969). *Play therapy.* New York: Ballantine Books.

Bratton, S. C., & Ray, D. (2002). Humanistic play therapy. In D. J. Cain and J. Seeman (Eds.), *Humanistic psychotherapies: Handbook of research and practice* (pp. 369–402). Washington: American Psychological Association.

Cattanach, A. (2003). *Introduction to play therapy.* Hove: Routledge.

Chazan, S. E. (2002). *Profiles of play: Assessing and observing structure and process in play therapy.* Jessica Kingsley Publishers. Retrieved from https://ebookcentral.proquest.com.

Coşkunsu, G. (2015). *The archaeological study of childhood: Interdisciplinary perspectives on an archaeological enigma.* State University of New York Press. Retrieved from https://ebookcentral.proquest.com.

Erikson, E. H. (1963). *Childhood and society.* New York: W. W. Norton & Company.

Erikson, E. H. (1972). Play and actuality. In M. Piers (Ed.), *Play and development* (pp. 127–168). New York: W. W. Norton.

Erikson, E. H. (1977). *Toys and reasons. Stages in the ritualization of experience.* New York: W.W. Norton & Company, Inc.

Garson, P. (2013). History of miniature: Tales told by toy soldiers. *Antique Shoppe Newspaper*, 26(12), pp. 19–28.

Homeyer, L., & Sweeney, D. S. (2017). *Sandtray therapy: A practical manual* (3rd ed.). New York: Routledge, Taylor and Francis Group.

Hutton, D. (2004). Margaret Lowenfeld's 'world technique.' *Clinical Child Psychology and Psychiatry*, 9(4), 605–612.

Kinnick, H. Q., & Wells, C. K. (2014). Untapped richness in Erik H. Erikson's Rootstock. *Gerontologist*, 54(1), 40–50. Retrieved from https://academic.oup.com/gerontologist/article/54/1/40/562408.

Kuttner, L. (2012). Pediatric hypnosis: pre-, peri-, and post-anesthesia. *Pediatric Anesthesia*, 22(6), 573–577.

Jennings, S. (1999). *Introduction to developmental playtherapy: Playing and health*. London: Jessica Kingsley Publishers.

Jennings, S. (2011). *Healthy attachments and neuro-dramatic-play*. London: Jessica Kingsley Publishers.

Jennings, S. (2014). Applying an Embodiment-Projection-Role framework in groupwork with children. In J. Howard & E. Prendiville (Eds.), *Play therapy today: Contemporary practice with individuals, groups, and carers* (pp. 81–96). London: Routledge.

Malchiodi, C. A. (2007). *The art therapy sourcebook* (2nd ed.). New York: McGraw-Hill.

Moustakas, C. (1959). *Psychotherapy with children*. New York: Harper & Row.

National Museum of Play. (n.d.). National toy hall of fame. *Stick*. Retrieved from https://www.toyhalloffame.org/toys/stick.

Rogers, C. R. (1957). Necessary and sufficient conditions of therapeutic personality change. *Journal of Consulting Psychology, 21*, 95–103. ISSN: 00958891.

Ryan, V., & Edge, A. (2012). The role of play themes in non-directive play therapy. *Clinical Child Psychology & Psychiatry, 17*(3), 354–369.

Schaefer, C. E., & Drewes, A. A. (2014). *The therapeutic powers of play: 20 core agents of change* (2nd ed.). Hoboken: John Wiley & Sons, Inc.

Sommer, M., & Sommer, D. (2017). Archaeology and developmental psychology: A brief survey of ancient Athenian toys. *American Journal of Play, 9*(3), 341–355. ISSN: 1938-0399.

Stagnitti, K. (1998). *Learn to play: A practical program to develop a child's imaginative play skills*. West Brunswick: Coordinates Publications.

Stagnitti, K. (2009). *Children and pretend play*. In K. Stagnitti & R. Cooper (Eds.), *Play as therapy: Assessment and therapeutic interventions* (pp. 59–69). London: Jessica Kingsley Publishers.

Turner, B. A. (2004). *H.G Wells' floor games. A father's account of play and its legacy of healing*. California: Temenos Press.

van Rosmalen, L., van der Horst, F. C. P., & van der Veer, R. (2016). From secure dependency to attachment: Mary Ainsworth's integration of Blatz's security theory into Bowlby's attachment theory. *History of Psychology, 19* (1), 22–39.

Wells, H. G. (1911) *Floor games*. London: Frank Palmer.

Williams, A. (2012). *FYI: What is the oldest toy in the world? Popular Science*. Retrieved from https://www.popsci.com/science/article/2012-01/what-oldest-toy-world/.

Winnicott, D. W. (1965). *The maturational processes and the facilitating environment: studies in the theory of emotional development*. London: Hogarth.

Winnicott, D. W. (1971). *Playing and reality*. London: Tavistock Publications.

Chapter 7

Learning to play
The art of science of pretence

Karen Stagnitti

Introduction

Play is the context for changes in children's developmental abilities. This is the essence of the therapeutic powers of play; that is, specific change agents are initiated or facilitated by play and this strengthens the therapeutic effect of play therapies for children (Schaefer & Drewes, 2014). The power of play itself helps produce the change. The power of pretend play has been demonstrated in studies by Quinn and Kidd (2019) and Creaghe (2019). Quinn and Kidd examined videos of 54 caregivers and their 18-month-old infants engaged in 20 minutes of play. The play session was divided seamlessly into ten minutes of functional play (that is, play with toys, such as a hammer and peg set, drawing and puzzle) and ten minutes of symbolic play (that is, play with toys, such as saucepans, teddy, cloth, cups, two blocks, toy phone and spoons). They found that symbolic play contexts, more than functional play contexts, facilitated the establishment and maintenance of joint attention between the caregiver and infant (Quinn & Kidd, 2019). Creaghe (2019) examined the videos and audio recordings from the Quinn and Kidd study for the same dyads when the infant was 24 months old. She found that the infants produced more complex language and spoke more often within the context of symbolic play compared to functional play. She also found that during symbolic play sessions, there was more conversational turn taking and the infants initiated conversations more often compared to functional play (Creaghe, 2019). Creaghe argued that symbolic play was a negotiation of meaning (teddy was drinking tea), whereas functional play was a negotiation of actions (e.g. hammer the peg in the hole). The results of Quinn and Kidd's (2019) and Creaghe's (2019) studies provide direct evidence of collective intentionality, that is, the negotiation of meaning where children understand the intention of the play (Rakoczy, 2008). Symbolic play is complex play, and the transformation of objects and actions need to be constantly negotiated (e.g. is the box a car or a bed) for the play to continue and for the participants to have a shared meaning.

Symbolic play is embedded in and is part of the concept of pretend play. Symbolic play is the use of objects in transformation as something else during play (for example, a block is a phone or a stone is a mirror). It is playing beyond the literal. Pretend play encompasses symbolic play and also includes the attribution of properties, reference to absent objects sustains symbolic thinking and decentration (for example, imposing meaning on a teddy as 'alive') (Stagnitti, 2010). Learn to play therapy (Stagnitti, 2021) aims to facilitate and develop the ability of a child to pretend in play. It is aimed at children who cannot or do not know how to play, for example, children with developmental delay and disabilities, children with autism spectrum disorder and children with learning disabilities. The underpinning theories and rationale in learn to play therapy are the cognitive developmental theories of play, particularly Vygotsky's socio-cultural approach (Vygotsky, 1934/1986) and person-centred therapy (Axline, 1974; Meador & Rogers, 1973). Within Learn to Play Therapy the therapist creates a zone of proximal development (Vygotsky, 1934/1986) where the child can increase in their ability to engage in pretend play from the level of play they understand to more complex play contexts. Vygotsky's theory is that learning develops within the child's social and cultural environment and capable peers and adults can extend the child's learning to more complex levels than if the child is left to solve problems within their own understanding (Vygotsky, 1934/1986).

Learn to Play Therapy begins with a play assessment of the child's ability in pretend play so the therapist has knowledge of how the child processes their play. In the early sessions of Learn to Play Therapy, the therapeutic skills of the therapist are modelling pretend play scenarios at the current level of understanding of the child. By engaging the child within the zone of proximal development, the therapist then engages the child through joint and focussed attention to play with the therapist. The therapist then uses repetition with variation to model to the child other ways of playing the same scene, for example, the 'tea' may be 'hot' or 'spilt' or teddy may like a drink. The child is then encouraged to go beyond their current developmental level until the child can spontaneously initiate their own play of 'having a cup of tea with teddy', thus the child has developed capability in play beyond their original ability.

The understanding of play development within learn to play therapy is akin to Vygotsky's view (1934/1986, p. xxix) put forward as development resembling geological layers in the earth's core. How children understand a concept in a play situation depends on how many 'geological layers' it is in and what role it plays, depending on the 'layer' that is activated (Vygotsky, 1934/1986, p. xxix). To be able to pretend in play within the child's social environment, a child needs to understand the intent of the adult or peer (theory of mind), go beyond the literal and understand what the object has been transformed into (decontextualisation), decentre from self and impose meaning on something or someone outside of the self (also required theory of mind) and understand the narrative of the play and roles of the other players. In Learn to Play Therapy, building the capacity of a child to be able to play also impacts on these areas or layers of ability (Stagnitti, 2021).

Rakoczy (2008) argued that young children do understand the imposed meaning in the play. Quinn and Kidd (2019) and Creaghe (2019) added evidence to Rakoczy's view by examination and identification of what abilities a child needs to employ to engage in pretend play with shared understanding with a capable adult (their caregiver). The social interaction between a capable adult and child is called role and dramatic play within Jennings embodiment-projection-role approach (Jennings, 1993). Her approach to play development is the embodiment and sensory play, projective play and then role and dramatic play with each stage overlapping, depending on the play of the child. This chapter focusses particularly on Jennings' role and dramatic play stage. As Rakoczy (2008) argued, pretending in play is 'collaborative intentionality' (p. 506). It is social collaboration with give and take to create a shared meaning between those playing (for example, Peter, 2003; Quinn & Kidd, 2019; Whitebread & O'Sullivan, 2012). This social aspect of play is explained by Jennings as role because role is 'the different sorts of behaviours that people learn in order to be fully socialised adults' (1993, p. 65). She aligns role play with dramatic play, particularly by four years when the child's play becomes complex with the creation of play scenes with the child and characters taking on social roles and fantasy roles (Jennings, 1993). Within role and dramatic play, the child gains understanding of themselves and of others as the child develops 'both an individual and a social identity' (Jennings, 1993, p. 68). Where the child's experience of role models is distorted, for example, absent, rigid or abusive, the child's sense of self becomes distorted and leads to behaviours that are socially not acceptable or controlling or reflect a distorted reality (Jennings, 1993). Jennings work is influenced by psychoanalysis, psychotherapy, socio-cultural development and Piaget's observations of intellectual development (Jennings, 1993). These influences led her embodiment-projection-role play therapy model to be concerned with the psychoanalytic, psychotherapy and social development of a child who is referred for behavioural or emotional concerns. In contrast, children who are referred for Learn to Play Therapy are children who do not know how to play or cannot play and have developmental delay or difficulties, that is, children identified as having social difficulties, including inflexibility with change and anxiety. As children develop their ability to engage in pretend play, unconscious emotional issues may be acted out in the play and the therapist then moves to combine co-facilitation with non-directive play therapy techniques in response to the child.

In this chapter, a young five-year-old boy called Jonathon (pseudonym) came to Learn to Play Therapy sessions with his biological mother.

Jonathon had been diagnosed with autism spectrum disorder, was attending speech pathology once a week and preschool four half-days a week. He lived with his mother and father and older sister. They were a loving family where both parents worked within a large regional town. Jonathon presented as a comfortably dressed curious child who was unsure of what to expect in this new situation. The first session in Learn to Play Therapy is the play assessment, which in this case was the Child-initiated Pretend Play Assessment (Stagnitti, 2019). I told him what we would do (the narrative of what would happen) 'We will play with these toys, then some other toys, and then I'll talk to mum and after I finish talking to mum, you can go out the door with mum to the car'. After this I focussed on the toys, showed him what I had, invited him to play with them and asked no further questions. I kept my physical distance from him, while still being able to observe his play. He became more relaxed halfway through the session. His language was limited and he engaged minimally in talk. He manipulated some of the toys showing repetitive actions and no logical sequences in his play. With the unstructured objects, he did relate the objects together in repetitive actions with no clear function to what he had made. He used one object substitution (the cloth 'thing' as a person). His play was pre-pretend with peek a boo occurring during his spontaneous interactions. His mum described a boy who needed to be given the full narrative of what was going to happen. This is not unusual for children on the spectrum as they lack a coherent narrative and are literal thinkers (Stagnitti, 2016). He did know how to use toys, for example, a truck can be pushed and animals can be taken for a ride, however he presented with no spontaneous sequences in his pretend play.

Synopsis of therapy process

In Learn to Play Therapy the therapist is a co-player with the child. In the early sessions, the therapist chooses play activities that match the developmental play level of the child. In choosing these activities, the interests of the child are taken into account as emotional engagement is important to therapy effectiveness (Stagnitti, 2021). The therapist introduces the play activity to the child and responds immediately to the child's responses. Playing beside the child, the therapist uses techniques such as modelling, repetition with variation, gaining focussed attention, emotional engagement and tracking the play. The therapist creates a safe and engaging space where the child's play skills can be extended and built (Stagnitti, 2021). This zone of proximal development is created by engaging with the child at their level of play, and then as the child begins to intentionally initiate their own play ideas the therapist challenges the child to a higher level of play. In the first therapy session Jonathon preferred to sit at the table and chop up the wooden fruit (this provided a physically smaller space with a table between him and myself). As he became more comfortable, I moved the play to playing shops with him being the shopkeeper and mum and I the customers. The role play was at Jonathon's play level as it was reflecting an out-of-the-home script which he had experienced. The interactions between Jonathon and his mum (Yvonne) and myself were stripped back to be simple, single actions to begin with, for example, the customer asked for an item Jonathon had in his shop. There was no exchange of money in this session but more a repetition with variation with each customer commenting on different aspects of the shop and asking for different items. He left happy. The next session he engaged immediately in building a structure with large blocks in the middle of the playroom. He was talking to the puppet that was helping him. During the construction, small dolls were introduced so they could live in the structure. One of the dolls fell and Jonathon 'fixed' the doll with a bandage. In this second session, Jonathon was relaxed. He used all the room and the play activities moved fluidly between construction, tea parties and playing doctors with two teddy bears.

Over the following sessions the play scripts revolved around in and out of the home experiences that he was familiar with such as cutting wooden fruit, cooking on a toy stove, eating and drinking and driving characters in vehicles. In the early sessions he joined with Yvonne and myself as we modelled the play as co-players. He didn't talk much. Slowly, his ability to spontaneously initiate and enjoy longer play scenes began to emerge. For example, he would move buses, take people out, put people in, drive them and create conversations between the people. I added a problem to his play by having my people fall down and he offered them a Band-Aid®. He also examined them and told me when they were well again. He played such scenes several times as he needed the repetition with variation to con-solidate his play ability.

During block building one session, he was very pleased with himself as he admired several structures, which were all different. I took Toucan, a large bird puppet, over to the construction and wondered aloud if it was Toucan's house and if a cloth could be used for a roof. He liked this idea, put the 'roof' on the building, put Toucan inside and looked through the bricks to see Toucan. He then put Toucan on his arm and began talking to Toucan who began to converse back to him. Then Toucan played hide and seek with Jonathon, and when it was Toucan's turn to count, he moved Toucan so Toucan couldn't see (decentration, theory of mind). He was now engaging spontaneously for 30 minutes in one play scene. As Toucan took on a life of its own, Toucan would become naughty and grab food which Jonathon responded to with laughing and smiling.

Jonathon initiated conversations between figurines who would encounter problems and express a range of emotions. His pretend play ability now included decentring from self (Toucan and the figurines were 'alive' and showed various emotions), object substitution (the use of symbols in play such as the bandage as a ladder), narratives with problems and resolutions (observed through longer logical sequences in play actions with imposed meaning and elaborate contexts for play scenes).

He began to say in sessions 'I've got an idea'. In response to his growing ability, I reduced my modelling of play activities as he now took the lead in the play throughout majority of the session. The play activities also expanded to include non-life experience events such as playing with a fire station. Following Jonathon's lead, we set up roads, fire station, houses (boxes) and a garage. He played putting out fires, getting the truck stuck in mud and figurines phoning, sleeping and eating sandwiches and pizza at their house. There was a logical flow to the play and he gave a verbal narrative of the play as he played. Object substitution was embedded in his play now, for example, he read a book to the fireman/figure using the block as a book and used a hammer as a crane.

His mother was a co-player in all the sessions and she supported his play by confirming his ideas and adding to them. For example, Yvonne and Jonathan had a dinosaur each. Jonathon said it was raining and he used a block as an umbrella. Yvonne copied Jonathon and put a block on the head of her dinosaur. As it was a brontosaurus, the block, which had three holes in it, slid over the dinosaur's head. Jonathon thought this was funny and laughed. Then he heard 'a noise', he took Yvonne across the room to a 'crashed truck'. He fixed the truck and together, he led Yvonne and her dinosaur to another part of the room to build a new cave for the dinosaurs.

Jonathon's play ability grew to pre-planning his play, initiating play scenes and developing the play narrative. To extend Jonathon's abilities further, I opened the toy cupboard and let him choose the toys he wanted to play with. On one occasion he chose dinosaurs which expressed several emotions. Jonathon produced voices for them and when they were coughing, he gave them medicine. Then they had hiccups! Finally, they had a birthday for several dinosaurs and also for Jonathon. As co-player Yvonne was insightful at adding problems and extending the play and responding to the character's emotions.

Jonathon's sense of self was changing. During one session, he wanted a box as a car for himself. One of the large doll characters put her hands out and measured him and then measured the car. This was to see how big he was so we could pick the box that he could sit in. He was so pleased. The large doll character and Jonathon then went for a drive in the car (the box), which drove through a storm (a big problem), and then had to be repaired. Jonathon was also recognising emotions in himself and others. In one session Yvonne was co-playing with him on the floor when Jonathon made a character very angry. Here is an excerpt from the play scene:

> Jonathon gently taps the fireman character with an object representing another person.

Yvonne whispers 'The fireman's sleeping. What's he doing? He's sleeping on the truck'.

Jonathon taps the fireman a little harder with a thermometer (the person). His character says in a gruff voice, 'Uuuuh, what's happening to me?'

Yvonne's character: 'Uh, he's in the red zone'.

Jonathon's character: 'UUUh'

Yvonne's character: 'Ohh'

Jonathon's character: 'UUUh, I still mad'.

Yvonne's character: 'Maybe I'll give him a cuddle'.

Jonathon's character, in a strong stern voice: 'No way!'.

Yvonne's character: 'I think he needs some space'.

Jonathon moves his character away and in a stern voice says: 'He was going away'.

Jonathon gets another thermometer from the toy medical kit, which is within his reach. His back now to his mother. He places the thermometer to his character's body.

Yvonne's character: 'Where are you going?'

Jonathon's character: 'I was goin' to make me better'.

Yvonne walks her character around Jonathon so that her character can see Jonathon's character. She pauses and observes Jonathon manipulate the thermometer on his character.

Yvonne's character: 'Yea, going for a walk makes me feel better sometimes'.

Jonathon's character: 'Yes, that's too hard'.

Yvonne's character: 'That's too hard'.

Jonathon's character: 'Yep. That's too h-h-hard'.

Jonathon continues to manipulate the thermometer onto his character's body. It is showing red with a sad face.

Yvonne's character: 'How are you feeling?'

Jonathon's character says, as Jonathon manipulates the thermometer to a smiley face (yellow): 'I is feeling very very happy'.

Yvonne's character: 'Oh good. I feel happy too'.

Jonathon explored emotions in his play scenes now, which incorporated more play materials. For example, one session he set up a scene with the car mat, two buses, five people, a petrol pump, eight black blocks, three boxes (houses) and nine animals. One of the people got very angry and so the other people didn't open the door. As a consequence, the person smashed the box house. The people escaped just in time when the police came and put the angry person in time out. The person settled down, came out of time out and all the people went to the zoo.

On his second to last session, the large doll character was the shopkeeper. He stood behind the large doll as she sat at the shop counter. He changed his voice when he talked for her and answered the phone for her (while holding the block phone to the large doll's ear). He took money for her and wrote receipts for the customers (Yvonne and myself). The shop ran out of items, so he would go to the toy cupboard (the supply room for the shop) and select more items for the shop. The shop leased a truck at one stage as there were so many items that needed stocking in the shop.

In his last session, he chose trucks, planes, kangaroos, octopus, roads, pirates, cannons, birds, boxes, whales and a bridge. He put out the blue cloth for water/ocean. He built a diving board from blocks beside the ocean and then green blocks for grass. Later the green blocks were surf boards for the people. He had a plan, he led the play with the characters interacting. He imposed meaning on the play, used symbols in play and incorporated absent objects. His play narrative involved problems and resolutions. There were even fireworks from the pirate cannon as he directed my figurine to lie down so it could see the fireworks. He chatted and talked for characters. He could plan, think out, set up and then narrate a story with various characters and events.

The therapeutic powers of play

The excerpt above describes the process of the Learn to Play Therapy sessions for Jonathon, with his mother Yvonne and I working as co-players. The process is now considered through the lens of the therapeutic powers of play (Schaefer & Drewes, 2014). Of the 20 core agents of change, nine agents are considered from the areas of 'facilitates communication', 'increases personal strengths' and 'enhances social relationships' as identified in Table 7.1 and will be italicised to easily identify them throughout this discussion.

The first powers to be considered are grouped under facilitates communication. Under this heading, *self-expression, indirect teaching* and *direct teaching* are included. Jonathon began Learn to Play Therapy with reduced language ability. He could not use language to express emotions or communicate through narrative. Through the process of Learn to Play Therapy, which

Table 7.1 Therapeutic powers of play activated by Jonathon through pretend play

Domain	Therapeutic powers of play
Facilitates communication	• Self-expression • Direct teaching • Indirect teaching
Fosters emotional wellness	• Positive emotions
Enhances social relationships	• Therapeutic relationship • Social competence
Increases personal strengths	• Creative problem solving • Accelerated psychological development • Self-regulation

facilitates a child's ability to spontaneously engage in pretend play, Jonathon increased in his *self-expression*, both verbally and non-verbally. As Jonathon played, he explored feelings, his figurines expressed emotions and he played out scenarios which paralleled his own life experiences as he explored solutions and consequences of problems. Play provides children with the opportunity to express their feelings and thoughts and to make sense of their experiences (Morrison Bennett & Eberts, 2014, p. 11). In his later sessions he was exploring feelings of anger and in his play he made his characters angry and expressed that is was hard to control anger, but after a walk his character felt very good. With his whole body immersed in the play, Jonathon (who had a diagnosis of autism) was able to articulate what his feelings felt like and how to cope with feelings.

Direct teaching, a therapeutic power of play, 'is a process by which the therapist imparts knowledge or skills through such strategies as instruction, modelling, guided practice, and positive reinforcement. The play therapist uses fun and games to capture children's attention and increases their motivation' (Fraser, 2014, p. 39). Emotional engagement of the child is paramount when Learn to Play Therapy sessions begin. This is particularly important as Learn to Play Therapy aims to engage children with no play ability to become interested in play. As Fraser (2014) notes, children do not initially choose to come to therapy. It is the skill of the therapist both to engage the child and to create a safe place and a feeling of total acceptance (see Axline, 1974) so that children do choose to continue to come. Jonathon looked forward to his sessions and was totally immersed during the sessions. Toucan the puppet and the dinosaurs assisted Yvonne and myself to support Jonathon in *problem solving* and continued engagement in building his ability to pretend in play. Modelling as we played with Jonathon is a key skill in Learn to Play Therapy and Yvonne and myself modelled play constantly during the earlier sessions. We would slide between Jonathon taking the lead in play and Yvonne and myself coming in to extend his skills in sequencing, object substitution and more complex play scripts. While Fraser (2014) discussed learning by example, in Learn to Play Therapy, the therapist plays beside the child as a co-player (*therapeutic relationship*) and while this shows the child how to use the toys in play, the ultimate goal is for the child to lead the play. Jonathan was leading the play throughout the whole session in his later sessions.

Jonathon initiated his own stories within the play. In this way, the power of *indirect teaching* was observed. Jonathon processed his feelings of anger through the dolls in the play. In his last session he also told the story of people who lived near kangaroos and the bush. His family were moving to a large property and in his play he carried out stories of playing in the bush and seeing kangaroos. In his metaphor and storytelling he was processing the changes that would be occurring in his life (Taylor De Faoite, 2014).

Under the area of 'increases personal strengths', *creative problem solving* and *accelerated psychological development* are applied to Jonathon's experience of Learn to Play Therapy. The engagement in pretend play brings with it the necessity to problem solve as characters in the play encounter difficulties to be overcome. Children can 'imagine different possibilities in play' and 'rehearse alternative solutions to problems' (Russ & Wallace, 2014, p. 213). Within his play, the cognitive and affective processes in *creative problem solving* could be observed as his character voices reflected stress then relief. He simultaneously used symbols in play as solutions to problems. For example, he used the bandage from the medical kit as a ladder so figurines could climb down and escape. As Jonathon developed his ability to play, his narratives became more complex and his use of object substitution was observed in every session. Using objects as symbols in play (such as the thermometer and temperature gauge as people), Jonathon had to laterally problem solve as well as create shared meaning in the play between Yvonne and myself. Over the Learn to Play Therapy sessions, the gap between Jonathon's abilities and those of his peers decreased. This leads to *accelerated psychological development*, another therapeutic power of play. Research evidence has shown the benefits of engaging children in play builds their abilities in *social competence, positive emotional* development, literacy and narrative, and cognitive development (Prendiville, 2014). Neuroscientists have shown the importance of stimulating play experiences and brain growth in children (Prendiville, 2014; Sunderland, 2007). Prendiville (2014) presented a case study of a child who underwent Learn to Play Therapy and the gaps between her abilities in literacy, maths, *social competence* and *self-regulation* and the ability of her peers were reduced. By the end of therapy, Jonathon no longer needed me or his mother to facilitate his play. He could generate ideas and carry out sequences which evolved into coherent narratives with problems that were resolved. His mother reported that he had friends and there were now few concerns about his entering formal schooling.

Play 'enhances social relationships' (Schaefer & Drewes, 2014). Children who can initiate and engage in pretend play have been found to be more *socially competent* than children who struggle with their play (Lindsay & Colwell, 2003; McAloney & Stagnitti, 2009; Uren & Stagnitti, 2009). Quinn and Kidd (2019) found that it was the context of pretend play, as opposed to functional play, that produced significantly more focussed attention and interaction between a parent and their 18-month-old infant. Creaghe (2019) found that, by 24 months, the same children were initiating more conversation and there was more turn taking between the parent and child when engaged in pretend play, compared to functional play. Children need to create a shared meaning with others in their play for play to be maintained (Rakoczy, 2008; Whitebread & O'Sullivan, 2012). As Jonathon developed his ability to pretend in play, his play scenes became more abstract. For Yvonne and me to play with Jonathon, he had to communicate with us the meaning of the play so that we could join him in his play. For example, when it was raining on the dinosaurs, he used a block as an umbrella. His mother understood the meaning of the block and also used a block as an umbrella for her dinosaur. This ability to communicate the meaning in the play also generalised to his home and preschool setting, where he could create meaning in play with others and also understand the meaning in his peer's play. He was able to play with others. He understood socially what was happening in the play. He was less anxious and was happier – life was good!

Conclusion

Learn to Play Therapy uses the principles of Axline's non-directive play therapy and Vygotsky to engage children who cannot play. Sessions begin at the child's developmental level of pretend play. The power of pretend play to increase children's self-expression, social competence, creative problem solving and accelerate their psychological development can be seen in Jonathon's development from a child who did not know how to play to a child who enjoyed play, explored emotions and was happy to build narrative and story. Yvonne, his mother, was empowered to play with her son and was joyful in seeing her child develop into a competent player. The research by Quinn and Kidd and Creaghe shows beyond doubt that it is the context of symbolic play (pretend play) that creates the need to establish and negotiate meaning in the play. Rakoczy's third way of collaborative intentionally (Rakoczy, 2008) adds more evidence to the therapeutic powers of play in creating ability in children to play. In being able to play, children like Jonathon experience a richer life as they can engage in play to process emotions and also understand shared meaning in play. The engagement socially with others is now Jonathon's to enjoy.

Recommended further reading

McAloney, K., & Stagnitti, K. (2009). Pretend play and social play: The concurrent validity of the child-initiated pretend play assessment. *International Journal of Play Therapy*, 18(2), 99–113.

Prendiville, S. (2014). Accelerated psychological development. In C. Schaefer & A. Drewes (Eds.), *The therapeutic powers of play. 20 core agents of change* (pp. 255–268). New Jersey: Wiley.

Stagnitti, K. (2010). Helping kindergarten teachers foster play in the classroom. In A. Drewes and C. Schaefer (Eds.), *School based play therapy* (pp. 145–161). New York: Wiley.

Stagnitti, K. (2016). Play, narrative, and children with Autism. In S. Douglas & L. Stirling (Eds.), *Children's play, pretence, and story: Studies in culture, context, and autism spectrum disorder* (pp. 51–71). New York: Psychology Press.

Stagnitti, K. (2019). *The child-initiated pretend play assessment-2*. Melbourne: Learn to Play. Retrieved from www.learntoplayevents.com.

Stagnitti, K. (2021). *Learn to play therapy: Process, principles and practical activities*. Melbourne: Learn to Play. Retrieved from www.learntoplayevents.com.

Uren, N., & Stagnitti, K. (2009). Pretend play, social competence and learning in preschool children. *Australian Occupational Therapy Journal*, *56*, 33–40.

References

Axline, V. (1974). *Play therapy*. Ballantine Books: New York.

Creaghe, N. V. (2019). *Symbolic play and language acquisition: The dynamics of infant-caregiver communication during symbolic play* (Doctoral thesis, Australian National University, Canberra, Australia).

Fraser, T. (2014). Direct teaching. In C. Schaefer & A. Drewes (Eds.), *The therapeutic powers of play. 20 core agents of change* (pp. 39–50). New Jersey: Wiley.

Jennings, S. (1993). *Playtherapy with children. A practitioner's guide*. Oxford: Blackwell Scientific Publications.

Lindsay, E. W., & Colwell, M. J. (2003). Preschoolers' emotional competence: links to pretend and physical play. *Child Study Journal*, *33*, 39–52.

Meador, B. D., & Rogers, C. R. (1973). Client-centered therapy. In R. Corsini (Ed.), *Current Psychotherapies* (pp. 119–165). Illinois: Peacock Publishers.

Morrison Bennett, M., & Eberts, S. (2014). Self-expression. In C. Schaefer & A. Drewes (Eds.), *The therapeutic powers of play. 20 core agents of change* (pp. 11–24). New Jersey: Wiley.

Peter, M. (2003). Drama, narrative and early learning. *British Journal of Special Education*, *30*, 21–27.

Quinn, S., & Kidd, E. (2019). Symbolic play promotes non-verbal communicative exchange in infant-caregiver dyads. *British Journal of Developmental Psychology*. *37*, 33–50.

Rakoczy, H. (2008). Pretence as individual and collective intentionality. *Mind & Language*, *23*, 499–517.

Russ, S. W. & Wallace, C. E. (2014). Creative problem solving. In C. Schaefer & A. Drewes (Eds.), *The therapeutic powers of play. 20 core agents of change* (pp. 213–223). New Jersey: Wiley.

Schaefer, C. E., & Drewes, A. A. (Eds.), (2014). *The therapeutic powers of play. 20 core agents of change* (2nd ed.). New Jersey: Wiley.

Stagnitti, K. (2021). *Learn to Play Therapy: Principles, process and practical activities*. (2nd ed.). Melbourne: Learn to Play.

Sunderland, M. (2007). *What every parent needs to know*. London: DK Books.

Taylor De Faoite, A. (2014). Indirect teaching. In C. Schaefer & A. Drewes (Eds.). *The therapeutic powers of play. 20 core agents of change* (pp. 51–67). New Jersey: Wiley.

Whitebread, D., & O'Sullivan. L. (2012). Preschool children's social pretend play: supporting the development of metacommunication, metacognition and self-regulation. *International Journal of Play*, *1*(2), 197–213.

Vygotsky, L. (1934/1986). *Thought and language*. (A. Kozulin, Trans.). London: MIT Press.

Chapter 8

Finding Sally

Discovering the self in role play

Carol Duffy

Introduction

I was fortunate to have been a student of Sue Jennings while training as a creative child and adolescent psychotherapist. In fact, the first play therapy text I ever read was her own 'Introduction to Developmental Play Therapy' (Jennings, 1999). So, to say her work has been formative is an understatement. Using Sue's Embodiment-Projection-Role (EPR) paradigm to track the process and/or assess my client's developmental and unmet needs became a bedrock for how I practise psychotherapy. The interweaving of understanding from the EPR paradigm complemented and blended effortlessly with Yasenik and Gardner's (2004) guide to decision making both in the micro moments of a therapy session and later in a reflective position, either on my own or in supervision.

The premise that our body is our primary means of learning (Jennings, 1999) resonates strongly in my work and is echoed in much of the neurobiological literature (Gaskill & Perry, 2011; Geller & Porges, 2014; Ogden & Minton, 2010; Perry, 2006; Perry & Pollard, 1998; van der Kolk, 2014). Indeed, I found the work of Bruce Perry and his neurosequential model of therapeutics approach (Gaskill & Perry, 2014) to overlap with EPR like a neuroscientific twin.

I am particularly intrigued by the capacity of role play to integrate and consolidate the three EPR domains. Role play is the third stage of development referred to in the EPR paradigm. The capacity to engage in role play refers to an individual's ability to take on dramatic roles themselves rather than projecting them onto other objects (Jennings, 1999). In role play the child is able to separate their play story from the reality of their lived world stories. The child can explore roles in different settings safely using dramatic distance (Jennings, 1999). This distancing and *as if* quality of the play allows the child to make use of their ascribed representations in the play and to paradoxically come closer to their actual story and confront and/or respond to it in a way that is not overwhelming to the child (Jennings, 1999; Norton & Norton, 2006).

In a role, a child can engage with their entire body. They can also project onto available props and materials any role, quality or emotion that they wish. They can connect fully and 'play' with complex dynamics and immerse themselves in a limitless number of roles. The child can choose a blanket to become a desert or a magic carpet to navigate one. They can cast their therapist in the role of a dictator or a submissive and frightened mouse. The child can become a powerful master or a rescuing hero. They can project onto the therapist, and materials in the playroom, a plethora of previously undigested and fragmented aspects of themselves and others as therapist and toys become their infinite blank canvas. In role play, the child can run, jump, roll, push, pull and climb – all during their method acting. Role play facilitates activation of the senses gently and with playful pleasure. This in turn soothes or awakens a nervous system into interactive engagement where oxytocin can flow through the body, promoting engagement and attachment (Whelan & Stewart, 2014). Space is created for a child's somatic experiencing of the safely distanced role and/or story where they are both the actor and director, facilitating a safer surge of the child's previously unexpressed and unwitnessed emotionality related to their story (Norton, Ferriegel, & Norton, 2011; Norton & Norton, 2006). The child can utilise all sorts of embodiment, movement and projection to release their cathartic expressions (Drewes & Schaefer, 2014), opening a unique window into their experiences (Norton & Norton, 2006). The child engages with embodiment, projection and role all at once when in role play, and they experience, and co-create within their therapist, moments of deep recognition and understanding. Untold stories begin to emerge and finally make sense. The child now has access to a witness, a regulated adult whose entire focus is intentionally geared towards co-regulation.

The playfulness and joyous nature that accompanies spontaneous and fluid role play creates fertile ground for the traumatised child to reclaim the sense of efficacy and agency which was once lost to them amidst the overwhelming nature of their painful narrative. Playfulness is the brains' greatest source of joy (Panksepp & Biven, 2012). I draw from the inspiring work of Teresa Kestly (2014, 2016) where she demonstrated a wondrous tapestry of therapeutic playfulness by blending the fruits from neurobiological and scientific discoveries on play with the broaden-and-build-theory of Barbara Fredrickson (2009, in Kestly, 2014). Fredrickson's work inspires the understanding that when we engage in joyful playfulness, our capacity to explore and allow characters in role play to try new solutions and share untold stories deepens, without the overwhelming aspects of the original assault. This facilitates much healing and re-patterning of our nervous system.

The safety that this creates coupled with new healthy feelings of empowerment, dignity and mastery lends itself to the prospect of a soothing and reparative experience (Geller & Porges, 2014; Norton & Norton 2006; Porges, 2017) as the neural networks associated with play overlap with those associated with healing. It is in this manner that a child can truly re-author and re-organise previously disruptive narratives and explore creative and healthier alternatives (Taylor de Faoite & John, 2011).

It is in this form of play that I have seen many 'firsts' (Landreth, 2002) and evidence of the four turning points described by Yasenik and Gardner (2019, pp. 18–23) as

1   'a change in thought, behaviour, affect, or understanding about something'.
2   'the emergence of a level of awareness not previously available to the child; something that is useful in the process of change either in a global or micro sense'.
3   'a moment in time where the child makes use of themselves or play objects in a way previously not observed, such as a change in the drive and direction of the play or the positioning of themselves in the play'.
4   'a change in what is illuminated or seen in the play: a change in the way of viewing self or others'.

Yasenik and Gardner (2019) suggest that, as these turning points emerge, the potential for the actualisation of the self becomes more possible and indeed visible. This was certainly true for the client, Sally, as presented in the following section.

Introducing Sally

Sally's birth mother concealed her pregnancy almost entirely, never connected with her baby and gave her directly into the care of substitute caregivers.

Sally experienced multiple placements, neglect and abuse during her early years until she was moved to her 'forever home' during her third year. Initially she was affectionless, meek and very quiet. By the time she was referred for play therapy at age six, she was described as pleasant and very much loved. Her foster carers reported huge tantrums in response to her merely seeing playful sensory opportunities such as sand or water play, and under reactions to stimuli that they had assumed would excite or create joy.

I was conscious that Sally had been exposed to a particularly disorganising set of formative experiences. She had not had a healthy formative experience of her body or a secure attachment experience where she could feel seen, felt, understood and safe.

When I met Sally, I observed a little girl who seemed desperately uncomfortable in her own skin. It looked as if her clothes were wearing her rather than the other way around. She did not engage with me directly and stayed almost entirely in one area of the playroom throughout her first series of play sessions. She brushed against/past my body several times in each session. Almost as if I was furniture.

Her presentation certainly demonstrated more anxiety than trust and suggested confusion over her body's boundaries. It was as if she did not notice herself against me (Jennings, 2014) or see me as 'other' in the room. While I have no doubt Sally was aware of me, her rigid and stoic gait suggested I was more likely to be generating a stress response in her rather than being a potentially available CARE system (Panksepp and Biven, 2012) that could soothe her in this novel situation. Furthermore, she showed no evidence of an activated social engagement system (Porges, 2017). Our social engagement system becomes activated when we feel safe. We detect signs of safety from others through subtle nuances in their facial expressions and facial muscles and through prosody in vocal tone. Not feeling safe takes us out of connection with others; it deactivates our social engagement system and prevents us from making use of the qualities that a safe relationship can provide. Even when the source of danger is removed the lived experience of not feeling safe can live on and can dampen the potentiation of a person's social engagement system. Creating safety in the context of therapy must therefore become a primary goal.

The initial treatment approach was to focus on building the therapeutic relationship. I paid close attention to the emotions and sensations that were generated in me (Norton & Norton, 2006) and developed a working hypothesis that this little girl's story was indeed locked in her body. Until her body became regulated and felt safe in contact with another (Geller & Porges, 2014; Kestly, 2016; Perry, 2006; Prendiville, 2017), active engagement in therapy would be a struggle for her and the implicit memories that she needed to process would remain locked inside, destined only to be told in a pained embodied way. The treatment plan was wholly focussed on safety (Porges, 2017). Play and relationship would be both the medium and the process (Geller & Porges, 2014; Norton and Norton, 2006; Norton & Norton, 2006).

The play therapy process begins

Initially Sally presented with high levels of play disruptions and fragmented play that was rigid and not joyful. Her persistent high stress levels and her struggle with playfulness indicated that she was on alert and highly anticipatory of a dangerous encounter (Norton et al., 2011; Schore, 2003). The spontaneity, unpredictability and even joy that play could potentiate along with greater engagement with another was something to be defended against (Fisher, 2003; Ogden & Fisher, 2007; Norton et al. 2011). Sally's initial perception of me seemed to be that I was a source of threat and not comfort.

I intentionally strove to communicate safety cues, bearing in mind the stage at which Sally's development was interrupted by negative experiences (Prendiville & Howard, 2017). Adverse childhood experiences (Anda, et al., 2006), attachment disruptions and relational and/or complex trauma

(Van der Kolk, 2014) weigh heavily on a child's ability to engage mean-
ingfully, communicate effectively and relate with others (Fraser, 2014;
D'Andrea, Ford, Cook et al., 2005; Perry, 2006, 2009; Stolbach,
Spinazzola, & Van der Kolk, 2012). It was clear Sally was wholly chal-
lenged in her capacity to make use of me as a co-player never mind as a
source of comfort. She felt compelled to defend against this. It was necessary for me to maintain absolute curiosity (Taylor de Faoite & John, 2011)
and total acceptance of her coping as necessary and valid.

I wanted Sally to know I was not in a hurry; I only wanted to know her. I
wanted to know her because she was *worth* knowing exactly as she was and
I tried to communicate this viscerally using non-verbal emotional transactions (Schore, 2003). I used a soft gaze, a warm look and a soft gentle voice
which I modulated consistently in response to her approach or avoidance
tendencies. I only entered the play when invited and resisted temptations to
interrupt with a therapist-led (Yasenik & Gardner, 2004) shift that my ego
suggested might move the therapy along faster. I used the dimensions model
(Yasenik & Gardner, 2004) to guide my decision making. Satisfying my ego
was not part of the brief.

While Sally engaged with sensory play in her first session, this was only to
show me her aversion and fearful response to it. She needed me to see how
painful and primal this body response was for her and thus indicated that
her struggle was rooted at an early stage of development when her sensory
play was not supported. Sally's body moved into rigid and defensive activation each time it had a sensory activation, and so being in the world was
extremely challenging as her body was simply not yet equipped for the daily
onslaught of sensory input she was receiving.

For the first two months Sally mainly used projective toys (P stage) which
were more controllable. She replicated the triune brain (MacLean, 1990)
beautifully but upside down in my water basin. MacLean's (1990) concept of
the triune brain is often referred to in the field of affective neuroscience
(Levine and Frederick, 1997; Sunderland, 2006) and subsequently psychotherapy (Prendiville, 2014) as a means to understand the evolution,
structure and hierarchical development of the brain. In Sally's projective work
I found myself confronted by the imagery that this model often generates:

- reptilian primitive creatures that may represent the instinctual brain
  stem area.
- mammals and/or domestic creatures that may represent the limbic and
  mammalian brain.
- human characters that may have represented the neo cortex and
  rational brain.

She tossed the miniatures into the water to ensure they or the water made
no contact with her skin. The mammals lay in the middle and the more

human symbols were buried under these at the bottom. She organised all the reptiles and dinosaurs to float at the top. This was the raw wound exposed and in need of attention. Her survival brain and its needs were at the surface and were almost unbearable to touch. Again, Sally was showing me how upside down her development had been. Her cognitive and reflective capacities were buried underneath a heavy load of survival and defence mechanisms. They were literally drowning under them.

As we moved into the fourth month of weekly therapy, Sally slowly but surely began to notice me as I matched and accepted her pace. I observed her to look my way, indicating a possible turning point (Yasenik & Gardner, 2019). I optimised my use of these micro moments to communicate unconditional positive regard, curiosity, interest and patience. Sally's rigid presentation began to soften, and brief but none the less real moments emerged where she smiled and we experienced genuine contact with one another, sowing the seeds for more positive relational resonance (Friedrickson, 2009, in Kestly, 2016; Oaklander, 1997).

I tried to convey to her the essence of what Paris Goodyear-Brown (2018) describes when she says 'I see what you are showing me, and you can show me more' using only my proximity and presence. I endeavoured to support a feeling of safety that could be experienced in an embodied way by Sally to invite further engagement and the potential to play freely.

I believe these were the foundational building blocks for what would become a bountiful and lush play therapy process whereby Sally could engage fully with the three domains of EPR and eventually engage with transformative play through the medium of role. Exemplars are used to illustrate the therapeutic use of role play as well as the activation of the four domains of the TPoP, which incorporates 12 of the 20 core agents of change throughout Sally's play therapy (see Table 8.1) (Schaefer & Drewes, 2014). In order to clearly identify the therapeutic powers of play, they will be italicised to easily identify them throughout this chapter.

The therapeutic powers of play in context

My playroom has many somatosensory play materials available, from small resources that can facilitate dry or wet messy or exploratory play to large body materials that facilitate whole body movements like rolling, swinging, rocking, bouncing, jumping and crashing (E stage). Over the first four months, Sally wove her way back and forth from small projective play materials and using only one tiny corner of the room towards tentative uses of these larger body-based equipment and toys. As her body experienced the permissiveness to engage at her own pace, her small steps became leaps and bounds.

From her fifth month, I began to see Sally running and jumping, exercising her body's capacities and expressing exuberance and pride in her

Table 8.1 Therapeutic powers of play activated by Sally through role play

Domain	Therapeutic powers of play
Facilitates communication	• Self-expression • Access to the unconscious
Fosters emotional wellness	• Catharsis • Abreaction • Positive emotions • Counterconditioning of fears • Stress inoculation
Enhances social relationships	• Therapeutic relationship • Attachment • Empathy
Increases personal strengths	• Creative problem solving • Self-esteem

newfound awareness of her ability to express herself in this embodied way. I observed how this play supported her ability to self-regulate (Yeager & Yeager, 2014). Sally demonstrated this in her intentional approach towards the use of materials that she had previously felt compelled to avoid. She appeared to now have greater capacity to manage her impulses and rather than continuous aversion and defensive strategies, I began to see more engagement and capacity to stay in contact (Oaklander, 1997). Sally began to engage with a formerly inhibited expression of her playfulness, a need to move and feel her body in a joyful way against something. She was clearly empowered and enjoying the release of her body's somatic surges in response to her sensory activation. Fostering and growing this potential within herself and the relevant, rewarding and repetitive (Gaskill & Perry, 2014; Perry, 2006; Perry, Hogan, & Marlin, 2000) patterning of this play in my presence *counterconditioned fears* Sally had previously shown. Sally repeatedly experienced the permissiveness and safety of the *therapeutic relationship*. Playfulness grew and she actively and indirectly practiced *creative problem solving* to manage her over-active stress response. Similarly, this facilitated *stress inoculation* against Sally's involuntary responses to me and playfulness in sessions going forward and in her life. Sally now was present in herself and in the relationship. I began to see her wear her clothes and not the other way around. Now she could begin to embody and play with other roles scaffolded by the therapeutic and strengthening effects of the therapeutic powers that were active in her embodied play.

A significant moment in the play came one day around 30 sessions into Sally's process, when she asked me to go down on my knees. Her body felt charged and full of its own potency and over time her rapport and permissiveness with me was more established and so was her burgeoning sense of security in this relationship. She did a jump and a tumble and then ran up on my knees and stood, as a toddler would, holding my hands and smiling into my face. I smiled back. In that moment I experienced a visceral shift whereby I knew something had changed. She felt my care and wonder in her and she enjoyed it. She enjoyed being enjoyed and was visited by a surge of *positive emotions*. I had stopped being a threat and became an opportunity and a source of joy and comfort (Norton & Norton, 2006). I noted a shared moment of transcendence where we both knew our relationship, and so her capacity to relate in general had escalated and we were now on another level. Playfulness underpinned and pollinated her attachment-seeking drive. This illustrated the therapeutic power of play related to *attachment*. It was from this moment, I believe, the capacity to reclaim and rewrite her previously untold story though role play was derived.

Therapeutic powers of play active in Sally's role play

Sally's play became more interactive, shared role play began as my involvement as a co-player was invited. She moved towards play with the tunnel and tents. I often note that when my clients use these materials, and even more so in combination with one another, they tend to role play scenes that are reminiscent of intrauterine and birth-related experiences. Naturally, no child can ever confirm this. But many children when using these materials will utter sounds very like those of a newborn baby. They will desist from using any word-based verbal expressions and rely on pre-speech utterances that either convey SEEKING or FEAR, PANIC/GRIEF initially and over time PLAY (Panksepp & Biven, 2012) and joy. This type of role play liberates their potential to engage with authentic *self-expression* that is not only limited to experiences they can freely access and recall in explicit ways. They can gain *access to their unconscious* and otherwise inaccessible body memories. As Crenshaw and Tillman (2014, p. 27) state 'Play allows access to the earliest experiences of the child that lie outside of awareness'.

Sally began to use both the tent and tunnel around her 35th session. For around three weeks she would hide in the tent and tell me that I was *not* able to see her and *not* able to find her. I was a lion who could not find her cub. I searched to no avail. She gave little to no direction other than to keep 'not being able to find' her. She did not direct me to keep searching but was explicit that the role was involved with 'not finding' her. She was in the role of not being seen or found. Within my role in the play, I felt uncertain, uncomfortable and slightly irritated. I did not feel in connection with her.

I was confused, lost and alone. I found I no longer enjoyed the game and wanted it to stop and be over. Internally I wondered how this related to Sally's mother's experience of wanting the pregnancy to be over. How did 'not being seen' relate to Sally's own lived experiences of being concealed, not being found, seen and/or connected with? The previously unrecognised and diffuse emotionality (Norton & Norton, 2006) that most likely related to Sally's first sensory experiences of the world seemed to be 'playing out' in her constructed role play scenario.

After three sessions of repetitive lost and not to be found role play, Sally began to burst out of the tent full of roars like a lion, yet across her face was stretched a huge triumphant smile and eyes that were bright with delight, thus portraying a primitive and embodied expression of *positive emotions*. If her body expression had words I believe it would have said '*Here I am, and I am proud! Now what ya' gonna do!?*'.

I was intentionally employing prescriptive activation of the therapeutic powers of *creative problem solving*; *counter conditioning fears*; *stress inoculation*; and attempting to kindle the potential for greater activation of the therapeutic power of *attachment*. I wanted the role play experience to activate her nervous system in an optimal and regulated manner, so she would seek further engagement and play with me. I wanted to expand the play and so her capacity to continue the repatterning of her neuroception and attachment seeking drives. The therapeutic powers of play (Schaefer & Drewes, 2014) accentuated and bolstered my clinical decision making and my immersion (Yasenik and Gardner, 2004) in the role play and the role play created the playground for this to actualise.

Non-verbal emotional transactions (Schore & Schore, 2014) were the means of our communication and I wanted to communicate to Sally that she was safe in this story. She had potency in this role and could emerge like a lion cub with a roar and expect to find a positive reception. She could now rewrite the story to be one where she was wanted and where she was not alone. Sally could reclaim fragmented aspects of her true self and embody them with *positive emotions* in this interactive role play.

Within another couple of weeks, Sally shifted the play again and told me to stand in the tunnel upright and hide inside it. I was then told to crouch down on my hunkers. Sally was laughing and giggling and attempting to hide behind me. It seemed she needed to be outside of my sight but not my mind at this point. Now it seemed as if there was no way she could be hidden! She then told me to jump up from my crouch and then leapt from her 'hiding' place behind me to position herself at my feet and again with peals of laughter she said 'I am a shark and I have just bitten you and now there is blood everywhere!'. I resonated with this play in a way that made me wonder about how it might be linked to Sally's birth experience. The content of the play startled me as I had never before had a child engage with this apparent narrative in such an explicit and almost gruesome way.

I wondered if this echoed a possible startling embodied and unconscious birthing memory that Sally was now able to engage with through her role play. I had no information about her actual birth and was wholly reliant on this felt experience between us as her means to exchange and share her unconscious story.

However, I utilised the containment of the symbolic play narrative to safely countercondition the stress response that was potential in us both and committed wholly to the play (Norton & Norton, 2006; Yasenik & Gardner, 2004). This allowed the *abreactive* power of play to remain active, further facilitated Sally's *access to unconscious* material and allowed her the capacity for *creative problem solving* in line with Barbara Frederickson's broaden-and-build-theory (Fredrickson 2009, in Kestly, 2014). This was the process of change in action whereby Sally's trauma history was symbolically re-enacted. She was now attempting to reorganise her perceptions and patterned response to the world. This is the essence of abreactive play (Prendiville, 2014) and Sally's ability to adjust, gain mastery and role play new possibilities in this story became possible and vigorous. Her body could now actively engage with implicit memories with dignity, mastery and potency to empower her whereas previously she was impotent. She also had access to an available CARE system (Panksepp & Biven, 2012) in me which she now could use due to the fact that her social engagement system had potentiated in direct correlation to the therapeutic powers of this transformative role play.

I trusted the process and I trusted Sally to lead. Sally in role as the shark, repeated this scenario many times in this powerful play session and each time I responded in role by saying how surprised I was to see this shark and how much I wanted to know her.

> 'This shark is doing an especially important job! Wow I am so surprised to see you there but now I am so glad to know who this is' 'It's you little shark! I see you!' 'It was you all the time'.

Emotional, right brain to right brain, nonverbal transactions permeated this play to create a healing *abreactive* and *cathartic* experience.

The shared joy we both experienced (Fredrickson 2009, in Kestly, 2016) also broadened the capacity for the story to deepen even further in the role play. *Positive emotions*, enabled greater activation of other therapeutic powers of play such as *access to the unconscious* and *creative problem solving*. The therapeutic powers were alive and complemented one another in a symbiotic and growthful manner through this powerful role play.

Soon after the shark session, Sally employed my skipping rope in a novel way. Each and every resource has the potential to serve as a prop and become inhabited by a charged metaphor in role play. So too did my skipping rope. Our prescribed roles evolved to resemble more human characters who had access to more words and cognitive framing. What had been buried at the bottom of the water basin was beginning to rise to the surface. She began to use a skipping rope and became both my captor and my saviour in a duplicitous role. The rope took on the dual characteristics of a lasso that could ensnare and choke me, yet simultaneously had the potential to save me and pull me back to safety. This felt hugely powerful and I reflected and validated both qualities of the rope. It was my hypothesis that the rope was symbolic of the conflicting qualities of the umbilical cord, her intrauterine connection to her mother. It had the potential to give her life yet at the same time was dangerous and toxic due to its lack of safe connection.

In this way, I believe Sally *counterconditioned fears* around potential caregivers. Her experiences both within and outside the womb had generated a disorganising conflict within her tiny body, teaching it that caregivers had the potential to give and threaten life in equal proportions. This lesson had been repeated in her early formative years. Research shows us that the impact of what happens in our first two months of life are the second most powerful predictor of our future outcomes, but that current relational health was the strongest predictor (Hambrick, Brawner, & Perry, 2018). For Sally, the ghosts of those first few months, layered by many repetitive traumatic experiences, had divorced her from the capacity to make full use of the current relational health that encircled her now. However, through her role play she had reauthored this story and shifted her perspectives accordingly.

Moments of positive resonance remained frequent during this sequence of play. I noticed Sally respond with intrigue and curiosity as I reflected the dual role of the skipping rope and my complex position in being concurrently dependent on and under attack by this rope. Her affect began to shift and signs of resolution started to appear. Over a few weeks, the rope became less dangerous to me in my role and I was assigned greater capacity to become empowered in relationship to it. Sally's expressed emotionality shifted and the direction of the play changed to include greater potential for soothing and safety. Sally became more empowered throughout this play and her playfulness soared, thus indicating another turning point. She was fundamentally different and there was evidence of an increase in her self-esteem throughout her role play. She also demonstrated greater *empathy* to my enacted character and even the rope was given credit for its central role, but nonetheless was made redundant. Her play began to show more and more levels of mastery, indicating a further turning point (Yasenik & Gardner, 2019).

Mastery play began to take the place of this role play and stories began to be told in Sally's review process that pointed towards an improved sense of self, *self-esteem* and comfort in her own skin. There was much less aversion to sensory stimuli and Sally began to play freely and joyfully with the somatosensory materials in the room including sand, clay and slime. In the past her sensory activation created too great a charge in her system thus priming her for defence and moving her out of relationship. Now she was able to enjoy it.

She could now engage freely, happily and relationally with these play materials. We continued to play together over a few more sessions until the end of her process. Sally showed evidence of increased personal strengths, her proficiency in the areas of communication, emotional wellness and the capacity to relate all showed marked and continued improvement.

Conclusion

When we draw from a humanistic and integrative approach that is trans-theoretical and intentional, we weave a tapestry of a therapeutic relationship that can traverse and uniquely respond to many complex and individual needs. Blanket approaches are not best practice when it comes to psychotherapeutic work with trauma, yet we do not need to be *ad hoc* either. When therapists integrate the teachings of EPR and marry these with the models of experiential play therapy (Norton & Norton, 2006) and the decision making guidance of Yasenik and Gardner (2004) while positioning ourselves firmly on the foundations of neurobiological discoveries, we can truly activate and exploit the transformative therapeutic powers of play.

Therapists can adopt a fluid, sophisticated and targeted approach that is child focussed, child led and entirely responsive and attuned to the hidden harm and unmet needs that have preoccupied and highjacked our client's nervous systems for so long. The above case example shows how the therapeutic powers of play incubated the role plays potential to activate the therapeutic powers of the play for healing.

> *Each individual 'hatches' and grows in a relational context, for better or worse.*
>
> (Schore & Schore, 2014, p. 181)

Sally certainly did hatch, in the context of relationships, and just like with the chicken and the egg it is impossible and perhaps irrelevant to try to decipher which came first. In this case was it the role play or was it the relationship? I believe that one generates the other in a fluid and co-operative interplay. The relationship facilitated the play and the play facilitated the relationship and through this union they gave birth to the active therapeutic powers of play, which then acted as the catalyst to cultivate the therapeutic process.

References

Anda, R. F., Felitti, V. J., Bremner, J. D., Walker, J. D., Whitfield, C., Perry, B. D., Dube, S., & Giles, W. H. (2006). The enduring effects of abuse and related adverse experiences in childhood: A convergence of evidence from neurobiology and epidemiology. *European Archives of Psychiatry and Clinical Neuroscience, 256,* 174–186.

Cook, A., Spinazzola, J., Ford, J., Lanktree, C., Blaustein, M., Cloitre, M., ... van der Kolk, B. (2005). Complex trauma in children and adolescents *Psychiatric Annals, 35*(5), 390–398.

Crenshaw, D., & Tillman, K. (2014). Access to the Unconscious. In C. E. Schaefer & A. Drewes (Eds.), *The Therapeutic Powers of Play: 20 core agents of change* (2nd ed., pp. 25–37). Hoboken, NJ: Wiley.

D'Andrea, W., Ford, J., Stolbach, B., Spinazzola, J., & Van der Kolk, B. A. (2012). Understanding interpersonal trauma in children: Why we need a developmentally appropriate trauma diagnosis. *American Journal of Orthopsychiatry, 82*(2), 187–200.

Drewes, A., & Schaefer, C. (2014). Catharsis. In C. E. Schaefer & A. Drewes (Eds.), *The therapeutic powers of play: 20 core agents of change* (2nd ed., pp. 71–83). Hoboken, NJ: Wiley.

Fisher, J. (2003, July). Working with the neurobiological legacy of early trauma. Paper Presented at the *Annual Conference, American Health Counsellors.*

Fraser, T. (2014). How neuroscience can inform play therapy practice with parents and carers. In E. Prendiville & J. Howard (Eds.), *Play therapy today: Contemporary practice with individuals, groups and carers* (pp. 179–198). Oxon: Routledge.

Gaskill, R. L., & Perry, B. (2014). The neurobiological power of play: Using the neurosequential model of therapeutics to guide play in the healing process. In C. Malchiodi & D. Crenshaw (Eds.), *Creative Arts and Play Therapy for Attachment Problems.* (pp. 178–194). New York: The Guilford Press.

Gaskill, R. L., & Perry, B. D. (2011). Child sexual abuse, traumatic experiences, and their impact on the developing brain. In P. Goodyear-Brown (Ed.), *Handbook of child sexual abuse: Identification, assessment, and treatment* (pp. 29–47). Chichester: John Wiley and Sons, Inc.

Geller, S. M., & Porges, S. (2014). Therapeutic presence: Neurophysiological mechanisms mediating feeling safe in therapeutic relationships. *Journal of Psychotherapy Integration, 24*(3), 178–192.

Goodyear-Brown, P. (2018). *Trauma & play therapy: Holding hard stories | Paris Goodyear-Brown, MSSW, LCSW, RPTS.* TEDxNashville. Retrieved from https://www.ted.com/talks/paris_goodyear_brown_mssw_lcsw_rpt_s_trauma_play_therapy_holding_hard_stories; https://www.youtube.com/watch?v=SbeS5iezIDA& t=203s.

Hambrick, E. P., Brawner, T. W., & Perry, B. (2018). Examining developmental adversity and connectedness in child welfare-involved youth. *Children Australia: Understanding outcomes for care experienced children, 43*(Special Issue 2), 105–115. Retrieved from http://www.cambridge.org.

Levine, P., & Frederick, A. (1997). *Waking the tiger. Healing trauma.* Berkely CA: North Atlantic Books.

Panksepp, J., & Biven, L. (2012). *The archaeology of mind: Neuroevolutionary origins of human emotions.* New York, NY: Norton.

Jennings, S. (1999). *Introduction to developmental play therapy.* London: Jessica Kingsley.

Jennings, S. (2014). Applying an Embodiment-Projection-Role framework in groupwork with children. In E. Prendiville & J. Howard (Eds.), *Play therapy today: Contemporary practice with individuals, groups and carers* (pp. 81–96). Oxon: Routledge, Taylor and Francis Group.

Kestly, T. A. (2014). *The interpersonal neurobiology of play: Brain-building interventions for emotional well-being*. New York: Norton and Company Inc.

Kestly, T. A. (2016). Presence and play: Why mindfulness matters. *International Journal of Play Therapy, 25*(1), 1423. Retrieved from http://dx.doi.org/10.1037/pla0000019.

Landreth, G. (2002). *Play therapy: The art of the relationship* (2nd ed.). New York: Brunner-Routledge.

MacLean, P. D. (1990). *The Triune brain in evolution: Role in paleocerebral functions*: New York: Plenum Press.

Norton, B., Ferriegel, M., & Norton, C. (2011). Somatic expressions of trauma in experiential play therapy. *International Journal of Play Therapy, 20*(3) 138–152.

Norton, C. C., & Norton, B. E. (2006). Experiential play therapy. In C. E. Schaefer & H. G. Kaduson (Eds.), *Contemporary play therapy*. New York: Guilford Press.

Oaklander, V. (1997). The therapeutic process with children and adolescents. *Gestalt Review, 1*(4), 292–317.

Ogden, P., & Fisher, J. (2007). The movements of play: Restoring spontaneity and flexibility in traumatised individuals. *Newsletter for the Global association for Interpersonal Neurobiology Studies*, Autumn.

Ogden, P., & Minton, K. (2010). Sensorimotor psychotherapy: One method for processing traumatic memory. *Traumatology, VI*(3:3), 1–14. Retrieved from http://www.sensorimotorpsychotherapy.org/articles.html.

Perry, B., & Pollard, R. (1998). Homeostasis, stress, trauma, and adaption: A neurodevelopmental view of childhood trauma. *Child and Adolescent Psychiatric Clinics of North America, 7*(1), 33–51.

Perry, B. (2006). Applying principles of neurodevelopment to clinical work with maltreated and traumatized children: The neurosequential model of therapeutics. In N. Boyd Webb (Ed.), *Working with traumatized youth in child welfare* (pp. 27–52). New York: Guilford Press.

Perry, B. (2009). *Examining child maltreatment through a neurodevelopmental lens: Clinical applications of the neurosequential model of therapeutics. Journal of Loss and Trauma*, 14, 240–25.

Perry. B., Hogan, L., & Marlin, B. (2000). Curiosity, pleasure and play: A neurodevelopmental perspective. *Haaeyc Advocate, 9*(August), 9–12.

Porges, S. (2017). *The pocket guide to the polyvagal theory*. New York: Norton.

Prendiville, E., (2014). Abreaction. In C. E. Schaefer & A. Drewes (Eds.), *The therapeutic powers of play: 20 core agents of change* (2nd ed., pp. 83–103). Hoboken, NJ: Wiley.

Prendiville, E. (2017). Neurobiology for psychotherapists. In E. Prendiville & J. Howard (Eds.), *Creative psychotherapy: Applying the principles of neurobiology to play and expressive arts-based practice* (pp. 7–20). Oxen: Routledge.

Prendiville, E., & Howard, J. (2017). Neurobiologically informed psychotherapy. In E. Prendiville & J. Howard (Eds.), *Creative psychotherapy: Applying the principles of neurobiology to play and expressive arts-based practice* (pp. 2138). Oxen: Routledge.

Russ, S. W., & Wallace, C. E. (2014). Creative problem solving. In C. E. Schaefer & A. Drewes (Eds.), *The therapeutic powers of play: 20 core agents of change* (2nd ed., pp. 213–224). Hoboken, NJ: Wiley.

Schaefer, C. E., & Drewes, A. (2014). *The therapeutic powers of play: 20 core agents of change* (2nd ed.). Hoboken, NJ: Wiley.

Schore, A. (2003). *Affect dysregulation and disorders of the self*. London: Norton.

Schore, J. R., & Schore, A. (2014). Regulation theory and affect regulation psychotherapy: A clinical primer. *Smith College Studies in Social Work, 84*(2–3), 178–195. Retrieved from http://dxdoi.org/10.1080/00377317.2014.923719.

Siegel, D. J. (2012). *Pocket guide to interpersonal neurobiology: An integrative handbook of the mind*. New York: W. W. Norton and Company.

Sunderland, M. (2006). *The science of parenting*. London: Dorling Kindersley.

Taylor de Faoite, A., & John, A. M. (2011). An introduction to social construction and narrative theories. In A. Taylor de Faoite (Ed.), *Narrative play therapy: Theory and practice* (pp. 11–25). London: Jessica Kingsley Publishers.

Van der Kolk, B. (2014). *The body knows the score: Brain, mind, and body in the healing of trauma*. New York: Viking.

Whelan, W. F., & Stewart, A. L. (2014). Attachment. In C. E. Schaefer & A. Drewes (Eds.), *The therapeutic powers of play: 20 core agents of change* (2nd ed., pp. 171–185). Hoboken, NJ: Wiley.

Yasenik, L., & Gardner, K. (2004). *Play therapy dimensions model: A decision-making guide for therapists*. Calgary: Rocky Mountain Play Therapy Institute.

Yasenik, L., & Gardner, K. (2019). Turning points and understanding the development of self through play therapy. In L. Yasenik & K. Gardner (Eds.), *Turning points in play therapy and the emergence of self: Applications of the play therapy dimensions model* (pp. 15–41). London: Jessica Kingsley Publishers.

Yeager, M., & Yeager, D. (2014). Self-regulation. In C. E. Schaefer & A. Drewes (Eds.), *The therapeutic powers of play: 20 core agents of change* (2nd ed., pp. 269–295). Hoboken, NJ: Wiley.

Part III

Connecting the four corners of the world of play

The therapeutic powers of play model in action

We metaphorically journey to the four corners of the world to delve deeply into the four major categories of the therapeutic powers of play model and examine the 20 identified therapeutic powers in real-life clinical cases. As we deconstruct the therapy process to better understand how play facilitates communication, fosters emotional wellness, increases personal strengths and enhances social relationships, stories of hope and repair will captivate you. Tales of Alex, Maddie, Danny, Bradley and Sammy exemplify the healing that is possible when the enzymes inherent in play are activated and aid in the emotional digestion of the residue of unresolved childhood trauma, struggles and distress. Play is both the medium and the process.

Chapter 9

Alex plays his unspeakable story

Facilitating communication

Alyssa M. Swan and Sue C. Bratton

In the second edition of their text, *The Therapeutic Powers of Play*, Schaefer and Drewes (2014) highlighted that one of the major powers of play is to facilitate communication, sub-categorised into communicative functions of self-expression, access to the unconscious, indirect teaching and direct teaching. Not only does play facilitate communication, play itself *is* communication. Major play therapy theories align with the notion that play is the most natural language of children and holds intrinsic value to the child (Allan, 1988; Guerney & Ryan, 2013; Jernberg, 1984; Klein, 1961; Knell and Dasari, 2016; Kottman & Meany-Walen, 2015; Landreth, 2012; Landreth & Bratton, 2020; Oaklander, 1988; O'Conner & Braverman, 2009; Schaefer, 2011). Play therapy provides the child with a therapeutic environment (playroom and materials) and a relationship with the play therapist in which to externalise and communicate their internal world through play. Because children have a natural propensity to express themselves through play over words, children's communication through play can be more spontaneous, instinctual and meaningful. Play also serves as a means for the therapist to enter into and understand the child's world and to communicate that understanding to the child. Play is the irreplaceable vehicle for developmentally appropriate and respectful communication with children.

At the end of this chapter, a case example illustrates the powerful and necessary role of play in the child's self-expression and access to unconscious desires and feelings, as well as examples of indirect and direct teaching. The authors adhere to a child-centred play therapy (CCPT) theoretical approach, thus the case and examples are presented through a CCPT lens.

Self-expression

Children are the keepers and communicators of their internal, emotional and perceptual worlds. Only through children's eyes can play therapists attempt to accurately experience and understand each child's unique world view; an honour play therapists are afforded when they fully experience children's play, free of anticipation or expectation for their playful expression. Landreth (2012) wisely declared that adults can only learn about children *from* children. In play, children are able to express themselves free of cognitive and verbal restrictions. Play is a universal language that allows children a safe and symbolic means to express feelings, wishes and experiences–especially important for children who are unable or have limited ability to adequately express themselves verbally (e.g. young children, children with communication delays and disorders and children who experienced pre-verbal trauma).

The various theoretical models of play therapy have similar but also distinct views regarding the role of play in children's self-expression. For example, cognitive-behavioural play therapists take a largely directive approach in facilitating children's self-expression through play (Drewes & Cavett, 2019), wherein the play therapist structures activities and play to elicit expression from the child typically focussed on the child's presenting issue. Adlerian play therapists encourage children's self-expression through play with goals of exploring the child's lifestyle, facilitating insight and teaching new skills (Kottman & Meany-Walen, 2015).

Whereas from a CCPT perspective, play therapists avoid directing or interpreting children's play, and instead wait for children to express inner experiences through self-initiated play. CCPT therapists attempt to attune to children's feelings, thoughts and experiences as children lead the play in order to understand each child's spontaneous expressions of self, others and their world. This nonverbal relational connection facilitates communication between children and play therapists. In the case example below, the second author describes how the child expressed himself through his play during play therapy sessions and during filial play sessions with his parents. An important part the child's communication was nonverbal and centred on his expression of his attachment needs–wanting to be close while simultaneously feeling hesitant to experience this closeness due to fear of abandonment.

Access to the unconscious

Several play therapy theories (e.g. psychoanalytic, child-centred, gestalt, Jungian) emphasise the important role of symbolic play to access the child's unconscious including implicitly stored early memories. In examining the role of play to explore and understand children's unconscious in psychoanalytic play therapy, Crenshaw and Tillman (2014, p. 28) emphasised that 'pre-verbal trauma can be resolved only through therapy that is not language dependent'. As shown in the case study that follows, the play therapist may observe the child repeating the same play behaviours as if they are compelled, particularly play that involves troubling experiences or trauma re-enactment from early distressing experiences that were pre-verbal or repressed.

Eliana Gil (2017) characterised this post-traumatic play as a sign of child resilience, children's 'efforts to process and manage traumatic memories' (p. 4) through play. Similarly, Violet Oaklander (1997) described the importance of unconscious regressive play as a celebration of children's essence and a means for the child to express needs that underlie the child's presenting concerns. From a Jungian play therapy approach, the therapist's primary goal is to interpret children's play to 'facilitate the process of making unconscious material conscious' (Lilly & Heiko, 2019, p. 41).

In the context of a child's felt senses of safety and trust within the therapeutic relationship, play offers a non-threatening window to the unconscious milieu of the child's internal landscape for both the child and play therapist to witness. In CCPT, play therapists trust children to determine, often unconsciously, when and how the therapist will be allowed to experience and enter into the child's personal world, which includes deep and often unconscious fears and intimate concerns. A child's unconscious navigation through play is illustrated in the case example during the phases of the play therapy relationship. As the child tested the safety and consistency of play, the playroom and the play therapy relationship, he no longer needed to rigidly suppress difficult and confusing memories. The non-threatening nature of CCPT provides a space in which children feel safe enough to be vulnerable through play to process and begin to integrate unconscious needs, desires and fears in a self-healing and self-directed way.

Indirect and direct teaching

The focus on indirect and direct teaching varies among the theoretical approaches to play therapy. Play inherently offers an avenue for indirect teaching to occur. During play, children can try out new ways of being, practise corrective and empowering actions and release restricted energy; lessons are indirectly acquired through spontaneous play. Indirect teaching through play can also include directive techniques including therapeutic storytelling, use of metaphors, bibliotherapy, co-constructed story making and play-based narratives to provide opportunities for the child to process emotions and express experiences and to practise and learn new behaviours and emotional responses (Taylor de Faoite, 2014).

Kottman and Ashby (2019) highlighted that Adlerian play therapists use play activities for the purpose of direct teaching during the third phase of therapy to help children gain insight through the use of co-created stories, playful activity and metacommunication. Drewes and Cavett (2019) described how cognitive behavioural therapists use play to deliver psychoeducation, teach coping skills, facilitate exposure therapy and systematic desensitisation and assess treatment goals.

In contrast, child-centred play therapists do not rely on indirect or direct teaching in sessions with children, instead allowing each child to direct the content and development that occurs during the play therapy process. From a child-centred perspective, relational safety and communication through play allows children an outlet for processing their experiences authentically, which therefore reduces their need to externalise their feelings through disruptive behaviours and transforms children's internalised self-perceptions to become more accurate and less restricted (e.g. 'I'm bad' to 'I'm worthy and lovable;' 'People will abandon me' to 'Some people can be trusted'). In play, children are able to naturally reveal new potentialities of their personality, spontaneously develop new coping strategies and freely explore new information and possibilities.

Child-centred play therapists may choose to incorporate indirect and direct teaching into relationships with parents and other caregivers, teaching CCPT attitudes, reflective responding and limit setting methods to parents during parent consultation sessions or involving parents fully in the play therapy process through filial therapy. In this case, the parents participated in child-parent relationship therapy (CPRT; Landreth & Bratton, 2020). CPRT is an evidence-based filial therapy model, which is typically delivered in a group format; however, individual CPRT is also viable and sometimes the clinically or practically necessary treatment option. CPRT contains three main components, including a combination of indirect and direct teaching: (1) therapists teach parents CCPT attitudes and skills during weekly meetings, (2) therapists facilitate group supervision among parents each week by viewing and discussing parents' video-recorded play times with their children and (3) parents facilitate video-recorded play times with their children, typically conducted at home (Landreth & Bratton, 2020). CPRT research demonstrates that teaching parents CCPT attitudes and skills results in significantly positive outcomes in their children's functioning (Bratton & Swan, 2017/2020).

Indeed, CPRT/filial therapy as well as parent consultation were important elements in Alex's successful play therapy experience. In the case example in this chapter, additional indirect and direct teaching activities were introduced to Alex's parents based on his readiness and needs expressed through his play during play therapy. Indirect teaching methods included providing caregivers with two children's books to read with Alex. Prior to the first play therapy session, a child's storybook on play therapy was introduced to lessen his apprehension about coming to play therapy by helping him understand what to expect. When Alex began to express through play his confusion and growing interest in his identity and being 'different' from his parents, a child's storybook titled *We Adopted You, Benjamin Koo* (Walvoord Girard, 1989), a narrative about late adoption similar to Alex's experience, was provided to Susan and Dave. Play activities designed to directly address specific concerns Alex expressed in play therapy are highlighted in the case example and include the following: (1) supporting Alex's adoptive parents in co-creating an adoption scrapbook with Alex to honor his early experiences and support his identity discovery process that he was working through in play and

(2) teaching Alex's parents *Structured Doll Play* (Bratton & Landreth, 2020, Appendix D), a story activity using stuffed animals and puppets developed to address Alex's worries about being separated from his parents.

Case example

The following case example illustrates play therapy with a young child, Alexander, who experienced multiple interpersonal traumas beginning before the age of one year. This case exemplifies the extraordinary power of play in how Alex, who presented with limited verbal communication, expressed his early and current experiences through play. The case is told from the first-person perspective of the second author. Identifying information has been changed to protect the child and his family. Alex was adopted from a Russian orphanage at four years of age and moved to the US with his adoptive parents, who were provided little information about his pre-adoptive experiences.

Alex was referred to play therapy at the age of six by his adoptive parents, Susan and Dave, after a school psychologist diagnosed Alex with reactive attachment disorder. Parents reported concerns about violent outbursts and refusing to be separated from Susan. Secondary concerns included eating and sleeping difficulties as well as speech and language delays for which he received services at school. Susan was especially concerned about Alex's 'rages' which often resulted in damage to their home and required physical restraint until he calmed down. Alex participated in play therapy and filial therapy (CPRT) for a total of 50 sessions over an 18-month period. Regular parent consultation and CPRT/filial therapy training were important components of treatment. As part of the filial therapy training, Alex's parents participated in 16 supervised play sessions with their child during the treatment period.

My initial objective was to establish a therapeutic relationship in which Alex would feel secure and safe enough to use play to explore and express his experiences, including pre-verbal experiences and those that in the past had been too threatening to admit to awareness. I trusted that in the context of a secure therapeutic relationship that Alex would direct his play in the way he needed in order to authentically express his deepest and most intimate concerns. I hoped to communicate through my way of being with Alex that nothing expressed in his play was too 'yucky' for me to witness and hold. I believed that a significant factor in Alex's progress would revolve around working closely with Susan and Dave to help them better understand how Alex's previous experiences impacted his current functioning. As they began to see the relationship between his early experiences, his unmet needs and the resulting behaviour that he chose to get his needs met, I believed that Susan and Dave would be able to accept him more fully. Because Alex was able to symbolically, and at times quite literally, express his world to them through his play during CPRT/filial therapy play sessions, they were able to grow in their ability to attune and respond to Alex's emotional needs.

Alex's first ten sessions were characterised by creating play scenarios to communicate his need for approval and affection by impressing me, by playing close to me, and by overt demonstrations of affection. In these early sessions, it became clear that no words would convince Alex that I already accepted him without condition. He would have to experience my acceptance firsthand before he could come to see himself as acceptable. During the fifth session, he used the flashlight to express his need to connect with me in a playful way. He turned off the light in the room and came close to me to shine the flashlight so we could see each other's faces, saying is his limited vocabulary, 'You; Me.' I responded, 'I see you; you see me.' He delighted – and the feeling was mutual – in repeating this game over and over, using self-directed play to communicate his need to connect. Themes of nurturing (sucking from the bottle) and trust ('being found' during hide and seek) developed during this period and continued during most of our time together. 'Hide-and-Find' was a favourite game that Alex delighted in. It was important to Alex that I ask each time, 'are you going to be easy or hard to find?' He was emphatic in his answer; communicating to me that finding him in the way he preferred was important to him. Because hoarding food and eating had become more problematic at home, I chose to include a healthy snack and a small pitcher of juice in the play room. He promptly poured juice into the baby bottle and began to drink from it. Sometimes he pretended to feed the baby doll, but mostly he used the bottle for his own nurturing needs. Alex's expressive language was very delayed and initially consisted of one or two word utterances; nevertheless, he managed to communicate his world to me quite eloquently through his play.

Alex's play during the next eight weeks seemed disorganised and chaotic. He was generally agitated and less focused in his play than in the first ten sessions. This phase was marked by the most intensely negative affect that Alex expressed during our time together. Alex persistently identified himself as a 'bad boy' and 'no good'. He seemed to be communicating through play and trying to make sense of early unconscious experiences of being abandoned and feel unworthy of being loved. For the most part, he abandoned nurturing and connecting play during this time. His play was often destructive and I felt that he was testing me to see if I would reject him as others had. It felt as if he was asking me over and over, 'Will you still love me if I'm bad/do bad things?' Again, no words could express to Alex that I accepted him no matter what; I relied on consistent relationship and unconditional warmth to communicate this to him. He needed repeated experiences of my full acceptance and unconditional positive regard before he began to trust that there was nothing that he could do or say that would cause me to reject him. Only then would he be able to grow in self-acceptance and experience himself as lovable and worthy of love. During this difficult period, Alex was showing me through his play that he was beginning to feel safe enough in our relationship to be vulnerable as he explored and expressed negative and repressed experiences and feelings, including his deepest fears and concerns around abandonment. He was on the journey toward healing.

The change in Alex's affect in our 18th session was remarkable. Whereas his play over the past eight weeks was constricted, agitated and chaotic, his play this week was spontaneous and joyful. It was during the last five minutes of this session that Alex first introduced the 'spinning game' he created that involved directing me to spin him around in a swivel chair while he directed me to touch and count his fingers and toes. Alex's play over the next ten sessions was characterised by greater spontaneity in self-expression and increased positive affect. During this time, he discovered the baby dolphin and chose it to become a central figure in his play. He often gently carried 'Baby' (designated a boy) around while he played, while other baby animals were thrown harshly into the sandbox, or he gave 'Baby' to me to hold and nurture, sometimes with a blanket. The spinning game, sucking the baby bottle, 'hide-and-find' and nurturing 'Baby' became almost weekly happenings throughout our remaining time together. The spinning game, in particular, became increasingly more intimate and communicative of his nurturing and attachment needs. He would often lie in the chair and suck from the bottle, gazing in my eyes as he had me gently rock the chair back and forth, and sometimes giggling while he directed me to spin him around and around and made up new games that involved touching. Alex had chosen a playful and safe way to deepen our relationship and work through his early experiences of what I guessed included inconsistent responses to his attachment and nurturing needs. Alex's play was clearly communicating readiness for attachment work, which needed to involve Susan and Dave through CPRT/filial therapy.

I met with Dave and Susan and we agreed to meet weekly over the next few weeks to discuss Alex's important attachment needs. We discussed how CPRT could be helpful and agreed to formally begin CPRT the next month. Susan reported that for the first time Alex was showing interest in what he was like as a baby. Previously he adamantly refused to acknowledge that he was adopted, saying, 'No! I was born in your [Susan's] tummy'. Based on Susan's report and my observation in play therapy, Alex was beginning to express interest in and confusion regarding his identity and being 'different' from his parents. I gave Susan and Dave a children's book, *We Adopted You, Benjamin Koo* (Walvoord Girard and Shute, 1989), a story similar to Alex's late adoption experience. I encouraged them to read the book to him if he showed interest. The book became his favourite bedtime story.

Around session 30, Alex introduced another significant play theme that continued for several weeks. His play was highly organised and purposeful. He began a ritual each week of putting the lit flashlight in the dress-up clothes trunk along with 'Baby' (the baby dolphin) and closing the lid. Before he left the playroom, he would open the lid to make sure the light was still on. Alex seemed to gain a great deal of satisfaction from his play during these weeks. Although at this point, I did not fully comprehend the meaning of his 'trunk' play, I understood that he was communicating to me that this play was meaningful to him, although perhaps on an unconscious level.

Shortly after, Susan and Dave began intensive CPRT training (Bratton & Landreth, 2020) twice a week for five weeks to fit their schedule and I continued to see Alex weekly. Alex played out some of the same themes with his parents that he played with me, particularly sucking from the baby bottle. During the pre-CPRT meetings with Susan and Dave, we discussed the idea that Alex might want to suck from the baby bottle or be rocked as an expression of his attachment needs. Dave was initially resistant to the idea that his now seven-year-old son needed a baby bottle. I explained that Alex may never have been held close and fed from a bottle like Dave had done with their biological daughter. We role-played how Dave could respond to such a scenario in a way that would convey his acceptance and encourage Alex to involve Dave in this play. Both Dave and Susan were motivated students and became proficient in demonstrating the CCPT play skills taught in CPRT. They delighted in the one-on-one playtimes with Alex. With supervision, they began to better understand Alex through his play. During this time, both Dave and Susan reported that this was the least stressful time in their family since they had adopted Alex.

During the play therapy session that coincided with the end of the CPRT training (session 40) and with five minutes left, I guessed that Alex had something important in mind as he blocked the door and taped it so 'we can't get out'. He quickly threw the clothes from the trunk and climbed inside with the flashlight. Then he told me to close the lid 'all the way'. To ensure that he was in control of his experience, I clarified that he would let me know when I should open it. He demonstrated that he would knock three times, and he did when he was ready to come out. During his fifth repetition of his important inside-the-trunk play and with one minute left, I bent down and whispered into the trunk, 'Alex, we have one minute left'. He immediately knocked on the lid to let me know he was ready to come out and ran over to get 'Baby'. He carefully laid 'Baby' inside the trunk on a soft piece of fabric, along with the lit flashlight and shut the lid. Again, I had no idea what all of this meant for Alex, only that his play was meaningful to him and expressed an important need.

Following this session, Susan and I met for our regular consultation. She reported that Alex had said the strangest thing to her this week: 'He asked me if he had a flashlight when he was in his other mommy's tummy'. Susan disclosed that this was the first time that Alex had acknowledged that he had another mommy. Now, Alex's flashlight-in-the-trunk play made perfect sense: He was trying to make sense of where he came from! Although he had previously refused to make an 'adoption story' as recommended by the adoption agency, through his play he was letting us know that he was ready. I recommended that Susan help Alex make an adoption scrapbook to help him understand his adoption story. I suggested that Alex be allowed to decide what should go into the scrapbook and we practiced how she could explain what she knew of his early experiences in Russia in developmentally appropriate words.

Session 42 marked new play that I believed were Alex's more overt attempts to make sense of experiences and feelings related to his abandonment by his birth mother and other caregivers, using an extension of his 'hide-and-find' play. The baby dolphin ('Baby') had long been a favourite and a meaningful toy for him; I sensed that he used 'Baby' to unconsciously represent himself. He took 'Baby', and with great care, buried 'Baby' deep in the sand. He abruptly left 'Baby' there and began to hammer nails in the log, which typically represented what I viewed as mastery play for Alex. I saw this behaviour as a 'play disruption' in response to his anxiety or discomfort (Findling, Bratton & Henson, 2006). Burying 'Baby' seemed significant to Alex, but he needed some distance from the play scenario and from his feelings connected to this play. Dealing with traumatic material can be re-traumatising; thus, it was important for Alex to approach this at his own pace. Towards the end of the session, he went to the sandbox and looked at me and said, shaking his head, 'Don't know where he is'. I simply reflected, 'Not sure where he is', not knowing who it was that didn't know where the baby was or if he would be found. I waited patiently to see if a story would unfold. After a few minutes of looking at the animals on the shelf, Alex chose the large dolphin (which I guessed might represent mother or caregiver) and a few other large animals from the animal family sets (which I later guessed might represent his multiple caregivers from his early experiences) and placed them in the sandbox. After I announced that we had five minutes left, Alex went to the sandbox and hurriedly moved the 'large ' animals all around on top of the sand as if they were all looking for the baby. Then, the large dolphin dug down and found the baby. Alex exclaimed with a smile, 'There he is!' He took the baby dolphin and made 'Baby' playfully flip up in the air. I reflected, 'It looks like he's happy that that one found him'. Although I was unsure who the large dolphin represented – perhaps his adoptive mother, Susan, who 'found him' in the orphanage or perhaps an unconscious wish that his birth mother or an early caregiver was still searching for him – but it was clear that he was happy to be looked for and found. Using animals rather than people figures to make sense of his early adoption experience seemed to provide Alex with the safety and symbolic distance he needed to explore and express his unconscious curiosities and implicit memories. Over the next few weeks, he played out several variations of this play theme of being searched for and found, sometimes including me in the finding, and always with great satisfaction of being found.

During parent consultation following session 44, Susan and Dave told me that they would like to go on a weekend trip to celebrate their anniversary, but that they had never left Alex overnight. We discussed Alex's readiness based on his progress in play therapy and at home and school. I reminded them about *structured doll play* (Bratton & Landreth, 2020, Appendix D) from the CPRT training and together we developed and practiced a story using stuffed animals and puppets to address Alex's worries about separation from his parents. Susan and Dave acted-out the story with Alex over several days prior to their weekend trip, with successful resolution of his separation anxiety.

Planning for the ending of therapy is important for all children, but even more so for children who have had multiple experiences of abandonment and loss. How I approached the ending of our relationship was critical so that Alex would not perceive me as yet another important adult who was leaving him. Because of Alex's developmental age, our long-standing relationship and timing (Alex's family planned a month-long vacation at the end of school), I decided that four weeks would be an appropriate termination phase. I explained to Susan and Dave that we would meet together next week after Alex's play session. I would be letting Alex know why I believed that he was no longer needed play therapy, and that I would ask Alex and Susan and Dave what they thought about ending our sessions. I encouraged Susan and Dave to say to Alex what they had reported to me about the improvements they were seeing.

During our termination sessions, Alex didn't introduce any new play; he engaged me in replaying our time together, both of us authentically expressing mutual delight in our relationship. Mostly, he enjoyed repeatedly playing his favoured hide-and-find and spinning games, with very little sucking from the baby bottle. When I went to meet Alex in the waiting room for our last time together he showed me the cupcake he had brought, along with a candle and small lighter his mother gave me. During our last session, he directed me to light the candle on the cupcake and sing 'Happy Birthday', after which he blew out the candle and said, 'Do it again!' Alex's birthday was a month away, but he seemed to have found a perfect way to celebrate our ending and at the same time, his beginning. We repeated the scenario 12 times, even after the candle was burned down. He looked into my face with a huge smile the entire time I sang to him. After the 12th round of 'Happy Birthday', he said that we could now eat the cupcake. Alex then jumped up and ran behind the puppet theater and yelled, 'Guess where I am?' I stood up prepared to search all around the room for him, when after just a few moments (not waiting for me to find him, as he had always done in the past), he jumped from behind the puppet theater, threw his arms wide in the air, and with a huge smile on his beautiful face, exclaimed, 'HERE I AM' I could not have summed it up any better! I responded by throwing my arms in the air and exclaimed, 'Yes, THERE YOU ARE!' I am always amazed by how children know what they need to bring closure to the therapeutic relationship if they have proper notice. Just thinking about our last moment together brings a huge smile to my face. Alex was free; he no longer needed me. He was well on his way to fully becoming all that he was meant to be.

Conclusion

Cultivating safe therapeutic relationships and listening to children's play allows play therapists to maximise understanding of and intervention in children's worlds. As depicted in the case example, play therapy provides the relational acceptance and opportunity for children to spontaneously and genuinely communicate their feelings and lived experiences through play. An important power of play (Schaefer & Drewes, 2014) is that play facilitates communication; this communication occurs during play by enhancing children's self-expression, accessing to the unconscious, and providing opportunities for indirect and direct teaching.

References

Allan, J. (1988). *Inscapes of the child's world: Jungian counseling in schools and clinics*. Dallas, TX: Spring Publications, Inc.

Bratton, S., & Landreth, G. (2020). *Child-parent relationship therapy (CPRT) treatment manual: An evidence-based 10-session filial therapy model* (2nd ed.). New York, NY: Routledge Taylor & Francis Group.

Bratton, S., & Swan, A. (2017). Status of play therapy research. In R. L. Steen (Ed.), *Emerging research in play therapy and consultation* (pp. 1–18). Hershey, PA: IGI Global.

Bratton, S., & Swan, A. (2020). Research evidence for CPRT. In S. Bratton & G. Landreth (Eds.), *Child-parent relationship therapy (CPRT) treatment manual: An evidence-based 10-session filial therapy model* (2nd ed.). New York, NY: Routledge.

Crenshaw, D., & Tillman, K. (2014). Access to the unconscious. In C. Schaefer & A. Drewes (Eds.), *The therapeutic powers of play: Twenty core agents of change* (pp. 25–38). Hoboken, NJ: Wiley & Sons, Inc.

Drewes, A., & Cavett, A. (2019). Cognitive behavioral play therapy. *Play Therapy*, *14*(3), 24–26.

Findling, J. H., Bratton, S. C., & Henson, R. K. (2006). Development of the trauma play scale: An observation-based assessment of the impact of trauma on play therapy behaviors of young children. *International Journal of Play Therapy*, *15*(1), 7–36. doi:10.1037/h0088906.

Gil, E. (2017). *Posttraumatic play in children: What clinicians need to know*. New York, NY: The Guilford Press.

Guerney, L., & Ryan, V. (2013). *Group filial therapy*. London, UK: Jessica Kingsley Publishers.

Klein, M. (1961). Narrative of a child analysis: The conduct of the psycho-analysis of children as seen in the treatment of a ten-year-old boy. *The International Psycho-Analytical Library*, *55*, 1–536.

Knell, S. M., & Dasari, M. (2016). Cognitive-behavioral play therapy for anxiety and depression. In L. A. Reddy, T. M. Files-Hall, & C. E. Schaefer (Eds.), *Empirically based play interventions for children* (p. 77–94). American Psychological Association. doi:10.1037/14730-005.

Kottman, T., & Ashby, J. (2019). Adlerian play therapy. *Play Therapy*, *14*(3), 12–13.

Kottman, T., & Meany-Walen, K. (2015). *Partners in play: An Adlerian approach to play therapy* (3rd ed.). Alexandria, VA: American Counseling Association.

Jernberg, A. (1984). Theraplay: Child therapy for attachment fostering. *Psychotherapy: Theory, Research, Practice, Training*, 21(1), 39–47. doi:10.1037/h0087526.

Landreth, G. (2012). *Play therapy: The art of the relationship* (3rd ed.). New York, NY: Routledge Taylor & Francis Group.

Landreth, G., & Bratton, S. (2020). *Child-parent relationship therapy (CPRT): An evidence-based 10-session filial therapy model* (2nd ed.). New York, NY: Routledge Taylor & Francis Group.

Lilly, J. P., & Heiko, R. (2019). Jungian analytical play therapy. *Play Therapy*, 14(3), 41.

O'Conner, K., & Braverman, L. (2009). *Play therapy theory and practice* (2nd ed.). Hoboken, NJ: John Wiley & Sons, Inc.

Oaklander, V. (1988). *Windows to our children*. Highland, NY: The Center for Gestalt Development, Inc.

Oaklander, V. (1997). The therapeutic process with children and adolescents. *Gestalt Review*, 1(4), 292–317.

Schaefer, C. (2011). *Foundations of play therapy* (2nd ed.). Hoboken, NJ: John Wiley & Sons, Inc.

Schaefer, C., & Drewes, A. (2014). *The therapeutic powers of play: Twenty core agents of change*. Hoboken, NJ: Wiley & Sons, Inc.

Taylor de Faoite, A. (2014). Indirect teaching. In C. Schaefer, & A. Drewes (Eds.), *The therapeutic powers of play: Twenty core agents of change* (pp. 51–68). Hoboken, NJ: Wiley & Sons, Inc.

Walvoord Girard, L. (1989). *We adopted you, Benjamin Koo*. Morton Grove, IL: Albert Whitman & Company.

Chapter 10

Polly meets Maddie

Fostering emotional wellness

Lorri Yasenik

> *My name is Polly and I am a puppet. I am five years old and I have ponytails. I like to play with babies and with the play food and the cash register and all the stuff in Lorri's playroom. I have lived in the playroom all of my puppet life. I have a special place where I sleep and sometimes Lorri wakes me up so that I can play with children who come to visit her. Some days I peek to see who has come to play. I want to tell you about meeting Maddie because Lorri said I could.*

Maddie's story

Three-and-a-half-year-old Maddie arrived for play therapy two weeks after being apprehended in the middle of the night by police during a drug raid in a downtown hotel room. Reportedly she had been found standing in the washroom while her mother was passed out on the bed. Two men, who were also in the room, were arrested and her mother was taken to hospital due to a drug overdose. Maddie was placed in emergency foster care and then later moved to regular foster care. While in her mother's care, Maddie's mother worked as a prostitute during the days and during that time she remained in the care of her mother's boyfriends (pimps). She was in her mother's care during the evenings. Upon referral, child protective services could provide very little detail about Maddie. Maddie's mother was mandated to attend treatment by child protective services and they disallowed any contact between Maddie and her mother.

Maddie attended weekly play therapy sessions that spanned a two-year period. During Maddie's first session she was verbally and somewhat behaviourally non-responsive. Beginning in a non-directive manner, I primarily used tracking and reflecting interventions. Half-way through the first session I became more directive as I began to pull out some dishes and play food and a baby doll and proceeded to play picnic. Maddie sat down and watched. She did not approach the play materials or enter the picnic play. I narrated my play scenario talking to the babies and offering some food and drinks to Maddie. Maddie watched and said nothing. I had many questions.

Did Maddie have age-appropriate play skills? What about her language skills? Was she frozen or immobilised? Externally, she did not appear upset or distressed, rather curious would be a good description.

Development and fostering emotional wellness

Prior to her arrival for play therapy, it was hypothesised that Maddie would at minimum be confused and disoriented. She had been in two foster care placements and had been taken abruptly from her primary caregiver by police in the middle of the night – with no further contact or understanding as to where her mother had gone. Previous to this she lived in an unstable high-risk environment. Still in early childhood, questioning and under-standing Maddie's development was paramount to thinking about facil-itating her emotional wellness. Was Maddie's development arrested from her accumulative life experiences? What should be considered prior to en-tering the play space?

In normative development, pre-schoolers demonstrate emerging language and communication skills, symbolic play ability, cognitive development (generalisation and thinking in categories, increased memory, increased awareness of causality), increased self-regulation (ability to imagine and anticipate consequences of behaviour), increased internalisation of moral values and self-monitoring and an increased sense of self that grows out of competence and autonomy. Hypothetically, what might have interrupted Maddie's normative development in these areas? Her mother's 'boyfriends' were the main caregivers during daytime. What was the likelihood that they were healthy, interactive caregivers who stimulated her growth in these areas? Might she have spent long periods without stimulation or was she often left alone? When in the care of the 'boyfriends' was she safe? When working with pre-schoolers, expressive and creative play-based activities are essential and are the primary pre-schooler language. We would have to wait and see what Maddie would show and tell through play.

When considering materials and activities for work with Maddie we must consider the child's presentation, growing abilities, and developing brain. Available therapy materials need to correspond to the child's drive to continue to develop gross and fine motor skills, sensory awareness, need for experiences with objects that allow for exploration, sorting and aligning, building, movement and music, real-life symbols such as food and cooking items, sensory and problem-solving objects.

Pre-schoolers tend towards magical thinking, which is a type of interpretation of reality through observing surface qualities vs. using reasoning. 'Magical thinking compromises accurate perceptions of reality' (Davies, 2004, p. 282). The reason puppets are so powerful for the pre-schooler to relate to the point that they believe in fantasy-based objects that move and act real (even if they do not look real) and in things they cannot see. Inviting Polly-the-puppet to come to engage with Maddie was an important decision. Children in this age group 'assimilate magic with the concrete reality of everyday experience' as a type of weaving process (Davies, 2004, p. 284). How would three-and-half-year-old Maddie come to think about what had recently happened? Would she blame herself for the disappearance of her mother?

Young children have mental models of their interpersonal relationships and these models shape how they view themselves and others. Fromberg (2002) has described social pretend play as partly driven by a child's internal schemas or internal working models (Bowlby, 1973). These schemas influence how children approach and negotiate their interactions with others during play as indicated through various play scripts. Affect tone (Kernberg, Chazan & Normandin, 1998) in children's play is a dimension of interpersonal schemas that is indicative of a child's worldview. Children's affect tone can be measured in children's play through representations of relationships on a continuum of threatening/destructive/unsafe themes to safe/positive/supportive themes. What would Maddie's affect tone be like? Would she use play objects in ways that demonstrate feelings of lack of safety and/or chaos?

Pre-schooler's emerging sense of self is related to a growing level of confidence and competence, autonomy, coping abilities, knowledge of sexual identity and racial identity. Additionally, children aged three to six are increasing their ability to categorise their experiences, which helps them to feel more in control and less vulnerable to anxiety. They are developing inner speech and private speech, which is used to sort experiences, rules and expectations. It would be expected that Maddie would need to feel control in the play therapy room in order for her to begin to feel more confident and potentially less anxious.

Maddie came to her second play therapy session, walked into the playroom and went over to the play materials and demanded all of the picnic items and told me to 'go get the babies'. She set the scene and directed the play. The power switched and Maddie was in charge.

What therapeutic powers of play contribute to emotional wellness?

Maddie, whether displaying symptoms of trauma or not, was viewed as likely needing help with gaining awareness of and control over distressing feelings. Six therapeutic powers of play assist in fostering emotional wellness: (1) catharsis, (2) counterconditioning fears, (3) abreaction, (4) positive emotions, (5) stress inoculation and (6) stress management (Schaefer & Drewes, 2014). Each of these areas will be defined and discussed. Polly agreed to assist in sharing some of what happened for Maddie during the play therapy process and how each of the powers of play contributed to her emotional recovery and increased emotional wellness. Polly not only observed things, she was a central play figure in the process. Polly will make some comments as to what happened between her and Maddie.

Catharsis

Drewes and Schaefer (2014) described catharsis as the storing of emotional distress that builds and is then expressed or 'vented' so the tension and the negative psychological experience is expelled, thereby allowing a person to gain relief. It is not the simple arousal of and then discharge of anger (for instance) that leads to resolution or a different emotional state; rather, catharsis requires arousal and then an exploration of its meaning (Bohart, 1980). Catharsis actions such as hitting a 'Bobo' doll, ripping paper, throwing objects, etc. requires therapeutic facilitation to bring insight and understanding. Play therapy offers a wide range of expressive materials and play objects which allows for cathartic play, which includes verbal, physical and emotional expressions.

Children may act out negative or traumatic experiences that have happened to them which in turn can lead to lessening emotional and psychological impact (Freud, 1920). Crenshaw (2015), when referring to *children of fury,* notes three stages of play therapy: (1) enactment of the rage, (2) displacement of the action play into symbolisation and (3) mastery of the rage through symbolised play. These stages all have cathartic features. For instance, indirect expression of anger onto a doll or toy object or character protects the child from any real-life retaliation from an offender but allows the child to do or say something they would otherwise not be able to do. Additionally, Schaefer and Mattei (2005) emphasised the point that physical play can cause release of muscle tension as well as negative affect.

Polly and catharsis

During the third session Maddie had been directing a picnic scene with the babies and I was assigned the role of 'friend'. After demanding I cook the food for the babies at the picnic, Maddie suddenly pivoted from the play and went over to the sandtray. Her back was to me and she just ran her hands through the sand. She suddenly disclosed 'Daddy Joe and Daddy Dave touched my pee-pee'. Spontaneously I decided to go to the puppet hanger and I chose a little girl puppet with a big mouth, ponytails and floppy arms. I woke 'Polly the puppet' up from her sleep and let her know that Maddie had come to play. Polly was curious and looked over at Maddie. Maddie looked back. I said to Polly 'something has happened to Maddie and it's just like what happened to you'. Polly said: 'Really Lorri?' and she proceeded to give Maddie all of the appropriate messages about telling about the sexual touching, how it was not right and emphasised her bravery. She also asked a few detail questions to try to anchor a bit more of what had happened. Polly told Maddie her age (five years) and what she liked to do. Maddie and Polly connected immediately. After this short exchange about what had happened to Maddie, Polly was put back to sleep in her puppet bed.

The next session Maddie walked into the play therapy room and demanded 'Where's Polly?' I woke Polly up and Polly became a significant figure in the room from that moment on. What therapeutic power of play did Polly represent? Polly will share her experiences of Maddie's anger and rage.

Polly gets hurt

It was really hard. Maddie didn't let me eat any of the food at the picnics. She gave me things and then took them from me. She used to hit me hard. Sometimes she ignored me when I asked her if I could play. She took toys and the babies away from me. She took things from me and gave them to Lorri. She would never share. She twisted my nose till I cried. She pulled my hair and told me to shut up and yelled at me. I tried to tell her she hurt me – but she just got more upset when I did that. She locked me in a room. She took a sharp sword and said she would cut me. Sometimes she was very scary and lots of times she was really mean. I think she wanted me to feel hurt. Lorri tried to help sometimes – like to help Maddie know when she was really hurting me, or to tell her about how I was feeling but for a really long time Maddie wouldn't listen to Lorri. I think lots of the things that she did to me must have happened to her too.

The projection of negative psychological feelings onto Polly occurred through most of our sessions together. There were times of relief, but mostly Polly became a character that potentially represented Maddie. Through Polly, Maddie showed things that likely happened to her while in the power of being the aggressor towards Polly. Although upset by it, Polly the puppet became an object onto which Maddie released her repressed aggression and strong affect. I did not encourage or lead the actions as is common in other directive cathartic play techniques (Cavett, 2010; Drewes, 2006; Goodyear-Brown, 2002; Kaduson & Schaefer, 1997, 2001, 2003). I did however provide a form of permissiveness similar too 'free associative catharsis', and Maddie's play behaviours could also be viewed as 'liquidating behaviours' where Maddie gained pleasure in the hurtful actions towards Polly, which later resulted in neutralising her strong emotions that were likely aroused by a series of specific life events (Scarlett, Nadeau, Salonius-Pasternak & Poute, 2005; Singer, 1993; Slavson, 1951). Parts of Ginsberg's four stages of emotional release in play therapy (1993) and Levy's three forms of release play therapy (1939) were present throughout the gradual mastery of her rage. Polly and I helped to increase Maddie's internal ego strength a little bit at a time. Titration was the act of slowing down Maddie's emotional and physical responses so that she could handle various competing feeling states. Polly helped Maddie to manage the speed of processing both historical and new experiences by intermittently approaching and challenging Maddie while also withdrawing from her and providing distance from uncomfortable feelings. Maddie was eventually strong enough to manage discomforting feelings and behave in a more pro-social manner. Relational repair became possible.

Polly the puppet witnesses abreaction

The term *abreaction* is regularly referred to in the trauma literature. Descriptions such as *re-experiencing play, post-traumatic play, abreactive play, trauma fragments re-enacted, revivication of past memories, memories previously repressed, re-enactment play, spontaneous abreactions, stored trauma* and *repetitive play* are all fall under the general term abreaction and are linked to trauma reactions and trauma recovery in the treatment of trauma (Ekstein, 1966; Gil, 2006; Goodyear-Brown, 2010; James, 1989; Nader & Pynoos, 1991; Prendiville, 2014; Steele & Colrain, 1990; Terr, 1983; Yasenik and Gardner, 2004, 2012).

During play, a child may begin by playing a scenario that appears to have a normative storyline and suddenly pivot from a role and act out a feeling state or another role that is out of context to the drama. What you observe does not seem to fit and there is usually a distinct sense that something does not make sense to the previous actions either in intensity or in literalness. Trauma memories can be stored somatically or in the sensory system whereby the memory of events may be stored in the more primitive somatic and visual regions of the brain (van der Kolk, 1996). It is possible for the limbic system to become activated while the verbal or narrative functions are not accessible. Re-enactment or repetitive play can be seen as an example of an attempt to work through a previous traumatic event. Without eventual interruption to assist a child to re-organise the scene, action, emotion, the child is left with a sensory and somatic level of processing that does not easily transfer to long-term memory and therefore interrupts the creation of a cohesive narrative of their lived experiences.

What did Polly witness?

I was playing babies and store with Maddie and she wasn't being as mean as usual. Then she did something that was not part of our game. She suddenly got up and went to the sandplay shelves and stared. She never uses the little sandplay things, so I didn't know what she was doing. I looked at Lorri, but she just watched Maddie. Maddie just stood there. I thought, 'I want to play'. Maddie surprised me because she picked up a little wooden cupboard with a door on it and brought it over and put it on the floor. That wasn't fair. I didn't want to play with the cupboard. It was too small for my baby or any of the pretend food. Maddie started to shake and she stared at the little cupboard and I got a bit scared. She started to yell in a scary voice at the cupboard and said really weird things. She said "no, no, not the guns, close the door, I don't want to"… over and over again. I was super mixed up. What was she talking about? There were no guns. Lorri put me down right away so I just peeked out while I laid there. Lorri said to Maddie, 'Its ok Maddie, you are here with me in the playroom, you are ok and you are safe, you are here. Look at me Maddie, nothing bad is happening now, nothing bad is happening now'. Then Lorri asked Maddie to touch her hand and she put her hand out so Maddie could see it. She took Maddie's hand and touched it really softly and she said 'see, you are here now and we are together and no bad things are happening right now'. Lorri held Maddie's hand and she said let's come over here (we have a big animal pillow) and we will sit together. Lorri told Maddie 'sometimes we have scary memories from a long time ago, but they are just memories and they are not happening again'. Maddie followed Lorri and started to listen. She looked really tired. I couldn't play anymore that day and Lorri just read Maddie some stories and I listened from my puppet bed. I didn't know what was happening, but now I think Maddie had a bad memory. Lorri said so.

Maddie's play behaviour appeared fragmented and was symptomatic of a literal re-enactment with much of the content occurring outside of her conscious awareness. Steele and Colrain (1990) may view this example as a spontaneous abreaction in that it was incomplete and uncontrolled. Maddie's body shook, her breathing was shallow, her face was flushed, the emotional intensity was high, and she was clearly frightened. What happened to trigger this play re-enactment is uncertain. It could have been any number of things. It is not so much a question of what triggered the abreaction, but how play therapists should respond. Grounding the child to the 'here and now', offering a short explanation as to what just happened and bringing calm and emotional restoration before ending the session is all part of the reorganising experience. I was a witness and responsible for assisting in meaning-making. There were numerous examples of abreaction during the work with Maddie.

Polly joins in on positive emotions

Positive emotions during play therapy fosters emotional wellness. This seems like an obvious statement, but what lies underneath this statement? If a child comes to therapy and experiences positive emotions, how does that affect their healing or overall functioning? There is much research in the area of positive affect, and according to Kottman (2014), who reviewed a body of research in relation to positive emotions, 'researchers have gathered data suggesting that positive emotions facilitate emotional, psychological, cognitive, physical, social, and behavioral shifts' (p. 107). In play therapy, many positive behavioural changes are noted through laughter, games, activities, positive regard, silliness and so on. Kottman, although frustrated by the question of having to explain what made positive emotions a therapeutic power of play, came up with a list of positive emotions sourced by her child clients. She notes 23 feelings that were exhibited through comments, facial expressions, behaviours such as hugs, smiles, humor and laughter and body language. Kottman states that no special objects or materials are necessary to evoke positive emotions but creating a safe space, being playful and fun yourself, modelling through expression of positive emotions are all critical to fostering emotional wellness.

The theory of 'broaden and build' (Fredrickson, 1998, 2001, 2003) refers to the ways that positive emotions broaden thought-action repertoires. The theory looks at how positive affect accumulates and incrementally impacts and transforms people towards being socially integrated, knowledgeable, effective and resilient (Fredrickson & Losada, 2005, p. 679). Research also supports the idea that it is difficult to retain a negative emotional feeling state when positive emotions are present or intermittently present (Garland et al., 2010; Teach & Lyubomirsky, 2006). There is some evidence that repetition of particular emotional states (positive or negative) will impact and potentially alter the function and structure of the brain. Tugade, Fredrickson, and Feldman-Barrett (2004) add that positive emotions mitigate negative health outcomes in both the psychological and physical realms. This can include interrupting depression and increasing positive attitudes towards self and others and increasing an overall resilient mindset. Interspersed into the play therapy process, positive emotions are essential to growth and development. It is more than happy moments or spontaneous laughter, or a game that has no purpose than pure fun, it is providing a dopamine wash to the brain that aids in recovery and actual transformation.

Polly joins the party

Lorri woke me up from my bed because Maddie asked her to. I was happy. That day Maddie saw the toy piano on the shelf. I love the toy piano. She tried all the buttons and every button played a different song. She liked lots of songs but she said: 'This one' and it was my favourite too. It was the 'happy birthday song'. Maddie said we were going to have a party. I was really, really happy so I asked: 'Can I come too Maddie?' Today Maddie was nice and she said 'ok'. Maddie said 'get all the babies' so I helped Lorri get them all. All the babies could come to the party because Maddie said so. Maddie put the toy piano in the middle of the floor and pushed the button. The happy birthday song came on and Maddie started to dance. Lorri and I started to dance too. We hopped up and down and twirled in circles. I got a bit dizzy. Lorri got the big fans with the silk scarves on the end and we all got one. We danced a lot and laughed a lot. Sometimes we bumped into each other. Maddie was in charge of the birthday song and every time it stopped, she started it again. The party lasted the whole time until it was time for Maddie to go home. The next time Maddie came, we did the same thing and the next time and the next time. I was really happy and Maddie looked really happy. She brought her baby from home. Maddie's baby's name was 'Smiley'. She was a really old dirty baby with no hair, but she came to the party too. We all took turns helping all the babies to dance. Lorri blew up balloons and we danced and hit the balloons until we got really tired and sat down on the floor and then we ate pretend cake.

Maddie spontaneously found the music in the room and initiated the theme of a birthday party. She had previously been intense and serious during play: intermittently abusive and harsh towards Polly and re-enacting scenes of rejection, control and food deprivation. The party theme infused new energy into the room, joined us as a social group and created a deeper relational connection. The positive emotions were contagious and I could see Maddie emerging in a more integrated way. Her sense of self and self-efficacy was palpable. The birthday theme may also be indicative of growth and development in a normative way in that the celebration of a birthday marks a special marker of arrival and acknowledgement. It is one way young children begin to understand the importance of their existence.

Counterconditioning fears: Polly the puppet wants the magic wand too

How do you assist children to reduce or extinguish fear and/or anxiety? Surely diminishing these emotional states leads to greater emotional wellness and the playroom is a safe place to assist children to take charge and have an empowering experience. Counterconditioning procedures come from the behavioural therapy specialists. Counterconditioning occurs when a fear response is paired with an opposite such as playing a game in the dark when a child is generally afraid of the dark. My playroom has always had a light that could be turned on or off, for instance, and flashlights are always available to manage fear of the dark in incremental steps. For example, imagine role playing being a space explorer on the dark side of the moon. The lights go out and we turn on our flashlights as we become secret agent explorers looking for a treasure. Play is children's natural way of communicating and games and play-based activities have the power of taking a negative feeling states and turning them into feelings of power, joy, excitement and competency.

Wolpe (1958, 1969) was a pioneer in the area of counterconditioning procedures. He was known for the now well-used 'systematic desensitization' process whereby he first taught a client to respond to their fear by utilising relaxation strategies, then to develop a hierarchy of fear from the least to most fearful, and then to practice relaxation while imagining the least fearful example first and then to continue on incrementally to the most fearful example. This gradual exposure helps clients to practice a competing response so that it becomes more available and more likely than the negative stimulus. Desensitisation processes for children are typically less cognitive and more experiential and play based. Magic wands, super hero capes, therapeutic stories and art-making activities that change the context of the fear such as 'emotive imagery' (Lazarus & Abramovitz, 1962), games such as making a plane out of boxes and becoming a pilot for child who is afraid of flying, puppets, bubbles, balloons, art materials and play weapons can all be facilitative aids for counterconditioning fears. In play therapy, the key is to be in charge of the fear. Externalising a fear by drawing the monster in the bad dream and then playing tricks on the monster or using a target shooting game to shoot at the image and then erase the image a little at a time after each shot are a couple of examples. Throughout the game(s), the child and therapist are making comments such 'you can't trick me' or 'so sorry you thought you were so strong'! Little by little each time the monster is re-drawn, it is drawn smaller with fewer details and less power. The power is returned to the child as the child is in control of the fear.

Polly the puppet, the wand, the sword and the spooky whale

Maddie and I were playing babies and food with Lorri. But Maddie surprised me because she suddenly went to find the play sword. She brought it back and said she was going to cut me – I was really scared and said so and I started to say I don't like it and it made me cry a bit. Maddie looked happy that she was making me scared. She ran to the play box and got out a wand. She said I wasn't here anymore and she put a spell on me. She said I was somewhere else – at the old house. I froze and then she used the wand to make me go to the old house. I was shivering because I didn't like the old house. Maddie went to the white board and drew something and I had to watch. She finished it and said it was a 'spooky whale'. It was really spooky. I was scared. Maddie took the magic wand and made another spell. She said that I was back now at this house and it was a nice house. I was happy. It was a nicer place. Maddie was kind of happy that I had to watch the spooky whale but then she was nice again when she said I could come back.

Maddie often used Polly to countercondition fears. In the example given by Polly, both the regression in time and later progression related to the old and new houses was apparent. Maddie was in control of the past emotional experience as indicated through the use of the sword and the wand. The sword initiated the fear in the play space through scaring Polly and then Maddie took charge of going to the past. She then drew an eerie-looking 'spooky whale' encapsulating a feeling state in the image. She froze Polly and made her watch. She then took charge of bringing Polly back into the present and more positive affect returned to the play. This was also an example of self-initiated titration (a slowing down of the system), which increases the possibility of integration of feelings and experiences post trauma.

Stress management and emotional wellness

If a child can play, they can use play to manage and often decrease stress. Bernard and Dozier (2010) note that play can decrease cortisol hormones responsible for the body's stress response. Maddie was driven during her play sessions to self-soothe and modify states of hyperarousal. She initially went to the sandtray and moved the sand around prior to making a disclosure of sexual abuse. Over the course of therapy, she continued to intermittently pivot from play to make contact with the sand. Once soothed by the texture, temperature and movement of the sand, she returned to the previous play actions. Sensory and messy play offer non-verbal (and verbal) opportunities for self-expression and increase body awareness and the emergence of self. Through soothing play, both hemispheres of the brain are activated, and rhythmic, repetitive behaviours assist in activating the regions of the brain which are responsible for self-regulation (Perry, 2009). The other significant example of self-soothing play was exemplified in Maddie's use of movement and music. She found the musical instruments and the self-playing piano and sometimes danced and moved for half of the session. Polly and I followed her lead and added to the rhythm and ritual of the dance. Rolling and rocking were additional examples of Maddie's play actions that increased her sense of well-being and relaxation. I rolled Maddie up in a big blanket and we often played roly-poly as she was rolled and unrolled in all across the floor. Maddie would laugh and ask for me to do it over and over again. Schaefer (2011) notes that laugher releases endorphins and reduces blood pressure and stress hormones. This being so, Maddie's system likely benefitted from these activities.

Fantasy and pretend play was a primary way that Maddie managed her stress during treatment. She was observed as spontaneously engaging with the play materials. On one occasion I purchased a new cash register. Maddie became pre-occupied with how it worked, but once she discovered its various functions, she moved into being a shop-keeper 'in charge'.

The shop-keeper theme, although a normative one on the surface, was used to gain control over Polly. Maddie used the cash register game to manage the stress of Polly asking her to share and to be an active part of the play. She both allowed and disallowed Polly to participate as a player in the scenario. She would at times respond in a calm and reasonable way and at other times she would become upset and appear overwhelmed by Polly's requests and questions. Reportedly, Maddie had been having a lot of trouble with peers in playschool. She was easily upset and could not manage peer relationships. She would hit other children, take their things and easily cry and tantrum. The social stressors were numerous for Maddie. Polly assisted by incrementally challenging Maddie by making demands other children in her midst would likely make. Not unlike issues that arise in counterconditioning, Polly attempted to challenge Maddie a little bit and then she would step back. Maddie's stress level during cooperative play activities appeared to lessen as she was able to incrementally accept the needs and wishes of another person through Polly. Decreased stress was noted through Maddie's breathing, tone of voice, body posture, facial expressions and overall increased calm approach towards Polly.

Polly – it was hard to be friends

When I met Maddie, I thought she was going to be my friend. It took a long, long time. She was mean and didn't let me play and she never shared. She would shake and get really, really mad at me. Her voice would get all weird and wobbly and she didn't breath and sometimes she cried or yelled. I just wanted to be friends. Lorri tried to help us get along, but it didn't work. She even brought us bubbles to blow. She told us about how to make big and little breaths so our bubbles were all different. Maddie took all the bubbles and used them just for her. I was really mad at Maddie and I wanted to smack her – but I didn't. One day I got really sad because Maddie hit me and pulled my hair and hurt me again. I told her in my big sad voice that I didn't like it and Maddie got super, super angry. She started shaking and turned around so I couldn't see her anymore. She told Lorri to tell me to 'stop it'. That wasn't fair because Maddie was the mean one. Lorri put me in my bed and Maddie said I couldn't play for a couple of times. It wasn't fair. Later Maddie said I could come back. She was a little bit nicer. Things got better. At the end we were friends.

Summary

Maddie's emotional wellness improved over time. Increased wellness was experienced through play and her relationship between the three of us: Maddie, Polly and I. Polly was an important figure in the reorganisation of emotional experiences for Maddie. Maddie presented as a traumatised preschool child who was abused sexually, physically, emotionally, psychologically and spiritually. Polly was an externalised representation of Maddie as well as a symbolic friend with whom she had to negotiate emotionally and interpersonally. I became the safe adult (friend and mother figure) who offered restorative emotional reflections and experiences. Earlier in this chapter 'affect tone' was referred to as a dimension of interpersonal schemas indicative of a child's world view and one way to measure change through the child's play (Kernberg et al., 1998). Maddie's initial affect tone changed from threatening, destructive and unsafe to safe, positive themes. Through our interactions and the power of play, Maddie began to experience her authentic self. She increasingly understood her emotional states and became more able to respond in pro-social ways with others.

References

Bee, H. L. (1992). *The developing child*. London: HarperCollins.

Bernard, K., & Dozier, M. (2010). Examining infants' cortisol responses to laboratory tasks among children varying in attachment disorganization: Stress reactivity or return to baseline?. *Developmental Psychological*, 46, 1771–1778.

Bohart, A. (1980). Toward a cognitive theory of catharsis. *Psychotherapy: Theory, research and practice*, 17, 92–201.

Bowlby, J. (1973). *Attachment and loss: Vol. 2. Separation*. New York: Basic Books.

Case, R. (1998). The development of conceptual structures. In W. Damon, D. Kuhn, & R. S. Siegler (Eds.), *Handbook of child psychology, cognition, perception, and language* (5th ed., vol. 2, pp. 745–800). New York: Wiley.

Cavett, A. M. (2010). *Structured play-based interventions for engaging children and adolescents in therapy*. West Conshohocken, PA: Infinity Press.

Crenshaw, D. A. (2015). Play therapy with 'children of fury': Treating the trauma of betrayal. In D. Crenshaw & A. L. Stewart (Eds.), *Play therapy: A comprehensive guide to theory and practice* (pp. 217–231). New York: The Guilford Press.

James, B. (1989). *Treating traumatized children: New insights and creative interventions*. NY: New York: The Free Press.

Davies, D. (2004). *Child development: A practitioner's guide*. New York: Guilford Press.

Drewes, A. (2006). Play-based interventions. *Journal of Early Childhood and Infant Psychology*, 2, 139–156.

Drewes, A., & Schaefer, C. (2014). Catharsis. In C. E. Schaefer and Drewes, A. (Eds.), *The therapeutic powers of play: 20 core agents of change* (pp. 71–81). Hoboken, NJ, New York: Wiley and Sons.

Eisenberg, N., & Fabes, R. A. (1998). Prosocial development. In W. Damon & N. Eisenberg (Eds.), *Handbook of child psychology social, emotional and personality development* (5th ed., vol. 3, pp. 701–778). New York: Wiley.

Ekstein, R. (1966). *Children of time and space, of action and impulse*, New York, NY: Appleton-Century-Crofts.

Erikson, E. H. (1950). *Childhood and society*. New York: Norton.

Fredrickson, B. (1998). What good are positive emotions? *Review of General Psychology 2*, 300–319.

Fredrickson, B. (2001). The role of positive emotions in positive psychology: The broaden-and-build theory of positive emotions. *American Psychologist, 56*, 218–226.

Fredrickson, B. (2003). The value of positive emotions: The emerging science of positive psychology is coming to understand why it's good to feel good. *American Scientist, 9*, 330–335.

Fredrickson, B., & Losada, M. (2005). Positive affect and the complex dynamics of human flourishing. *American Psychologist, 60*(7), 678–686.

Freud, S. (1920). *Beyond the pleasure principle*. London: Hogarth Press.

Fromberg, D. P. (2002). *Play and meaning in early childhood education*. Boston: Allyn & Bacon.

Garland, E., Fredrickson, B., Kring, A., Johnson, D., Meyer, P., & Penn, D. (2010). Upward spirals of positive emotions counter downward spirals of negativity: Insights from the broaden-and-build theory and affective neuroscience on the treatment of emotional dysfunctions and deficits in psychopathology. *Clinical Psychology Review, 30*, 849–864.

Gil, E. (2006). *Helping abused and traumatized children: Integrating directive and non-directive approaches*. New York, NY: Guilford Press.

Ginsberg, B. G. (1993). Catharsis. In C. E. Schaefer (Ed.), *The therapeutic powers of play* (pp. 107–114). Northvale, NJ: Aronson.

Goodyear-Brown, P. (2002). *Digging for buried treasure 2: Another 52 prop-based play therapy interventions for treating the problems of childhood*. Nashville, TN: Paris Goodyear-Brown.

Goodyear-Brown, P. (2010). *Play therapy with traumatized children: A prescriptive approach*. Hoboken, NJ: Wiley.

Kaduson, H. G., & Schaefer, C. E. (2003). *101 favorite play therapy techniques* (Vol. III). Northvale, NJ: Aronson.

Kernberg, P., Chazan, S. E., & Normandin, L. (1998). The children's play therapy instrument (CPTI): Description development and reliability studies. *The Journal of Psychotherapy Practice and Research, 7*(3), 196–207.

Kohlberg, L. (1984). *Essays on moral development: Vol. 2. The psychology of moral development*. New York: Harper and Row.

Kottman, T. (2014). Positive emotions. In C. E. Schaefer and Drewes, A. (Eds.), *The therapeutic powers of play: 20 core agents of change* (2nd ed., pp. 103–120). Hoboken, NJ, New York: Wiley and Sons.

Lazarus, A., & Abramovitz, A. (1962). The use of 'Emotive Imagery' in the treatment of childrens' phobias. *British Journal of Psychiatry, 108*, 191–195.

Levy, D. M. (1959). Release therapy. *American Journal of Orthopsychiatry, 9*, 713–736.

Nader, K. O., & Pynoos, R. S. (1991). Play and drawing: Techniques as tools for interviewing traumatized children. In C. E. Schaefer, K. Gitlin, & A. Sandrgund (Eds.), *Play diagnosis, and assessment* (pp. 375–389). New York, NY: Wiley.

Perry, B. D., (2006). Applying principles of neurodevelopment to clinical work with maltreated and traumatized children. In N. B. Webb (Ed.), *Working with traumatized youth in child welfare* (pp. 27–52). New York: Guilford Press.

Perry, B. D. (2009). Examining child maltreatment through a neurodevelopmental lens: Clinical applications of the neurosequential model of therapeutics. *Journal of Loss and Trauma, 14*, 240–255.

Perry, B. D., Hogan, L., & Marlin. S. J. (2000). *Curiosity, pleasure and play: A neurodevelopmental perspective. Haaeyc Advocate*, 9–12.

Perry, B. D., Pollard, R., Blakely, T., Baker, W., Vigilante, D. (1995). Childhood trauma, the neurobiology of adaptation and 'use-dependent' development of the brain: how 'state: become traits'. *Infant Mental Health Journal, 16*(4), 271–291.

Prendiville, E. (2014). Abreaction. In C. E. Schaefer and Drewes, A. (Eds.), *The therapeutic powers of play: 20 core agents of change* (2nd ed., pp. 83–102). Hoboken, NJ, New York: Wiley and Sons.

Scarlett, G., Nadeau, S., Salonius-Pasternak, D., & Poute, I. (2005). *Children's play*. Thousand Oaks, CA: Sage.

Schaefer, C. E. (2011). The importance of the fun factor in play therapy. *Play Therapy, 6*(3), 16–19.

Schaefer, C. E. and Drewes, A. (Eds.). (2014). *The therapeutic powers of play: 20 core agents of change*(2nd ed.). Hoboken, NJ, New York: Wiley and Sons.

Schaefer, C. E., & Mattei, D. (2005). Catharsis: Effectiveness in children's aggression. *International Journal of Play Therapy, 14*(2), 103–109.

Schore, R. (1997). Rethinking the brain: New insights into early development. *Summary from conference: Brain development in young children: New frontiers for research, policy and practice*. New York: Families and Work Institute.

Singer, J. L. (1993). Imaginative play and adaptive development. In J. H. Goldstein (Ed.), *Toys, play and child development* (pp. 6–26). Cambridge, UK: Cambridge University Press.

Slavson, S. R. (1951). Catharsis in group psychotherapy. *Psychoanalytic Review, 38*, 39–52.

Steele, K., & Colrain, J. (1990). Abreactive work with sexual abuse survivors: Concepts and techniques. In M. A. Hunter (Ed.), *The sexually abused male: Volume 2, Applications of treatment strategies* (pp. 1–55). Lexington, MA: Lexington Books.

Teach, C., & Lyubomirsky, S. (2006). How do people pursue happiness? Relating personality, happiness-increasing strategies, and well-being. *Journal of Happiness Studies, 7*, 183–225.

Terr, L. (1983). Play therapy and psychic trauma: A preliminary report. In C. E. Schaefer, & K. J. O'Connor (Eds.), *Handbook of play therapy* (pp. 308–319). New York, NY: Wiley.

Teitelbaum, J. (2006). Joy-based healing: 'A smile a day keeps the doctor away.' *Total Health, 28*, 59–61.

Tugade, M., Fredrickson, B., & Feldman-Barrett, L. (2004). Psychological resilience and positive emotional granularity: Examining the benefits of positive emotions on coping and health. *Journal of Personality, 72*(6), 1161–1190.

van der Kolk, B. A. (1996). The complexity of adaptation to trauma: Self-regulation, stimulus discrimination, and characterological development. In B. A. van der Kolk, A. C. McFarlane, L. Weisaeth (Eds.), *Traumatic stress: The effects of overwhelming experience on mind, body, and society* (pp. 182–213). New York, NY: The Guilford Press.

Wolpe, J. (1958). *Psychotherapy by reciprocal inhibition*. Stanford, C.A.: Stanford University Press.

Wolpe, J. (1969). *The practice of behavioral therapy*. New York, NY: Pergamon Press.

Yasenik, L., & Gardner, K. (2004). *Play therapy dimensions model: A decision-making model for play therapists*, Alberta, Canada: Rocky Mountain Play Therapy Institute.

Yasenik L., & Gardner, K. (2012). *Play therapy dimensions model: A decision-making model for play therapists*. London, UK: Jessica Kingsley.

Chapter 11

Sammy and the three-legged cat

Enhancing social relationships

Ken Gardner

Introduction

I was exposed to the therapeutic powers of play over 30 years ago, long before I became a psychologist and trained in play therapy. This exposure occurred when I was asked to spend a summer 'playing' with a four-year-old boy with complex medical and developmental issues including seizures, speech and language difficulties and motor-planning issues. This very endearing young boy, Bradley, was connected to a multi-disciplinary team at a local children's hospital. I was a teacher at the intensive day program Bradley attended as part of hospital services. Due to the frequent nature of his seizures Bradley spent most of his day wearing a helmet and was often too exhausted to actively participate in the program. Bradley's play was very fragmented and largely contained within the sensory-motor or the Embodiment (E) stage (Jennings, 1990). Although the program was goal focussed, I was simply given the directive to 'play'. In retrospect, this vague goal gave me no guidance for working, but with this directive came permission to find ways to engage and playfully meet Bradley where he was at developmentally. When Bradley returned to the program at the end of the summer team members asked, '*What happened? Is this the same child?*' Of course, he was, and of course I couldn't adequately explain what happened beyond stating, '*We had fun playing each day*'. I am the first to admit this is not the way to organise therapy; it took me another decade to figure out what happened!

Vignettes from my experience with Bradley will be used to explore the four sub-categories within the enhances social relationships domain. Through the case of a six-year-old boy named Sammy, I will then examine how these factors – therapeutic relationship, attachment, social competence and empathy, which have been carefully studied by neuroscientists and developmental researchers – are activated within the play therapy process.

Therapeutic relationship

Although I struggled to understand the potency of this change mechanism, and how best to activate it, this did not deter Bradley from eagerly anticipating when I arrived each day with a bag of select objects. Neuroscience research would suggest that Bradley was emotionally engaged by my playful invitations and experienced an increase in oxytocin, which engenders feelings of emotional well-being and trust. Our play-based interactions also activated mirror neurons, which helped me resonate with Bradley's emotional states (no wonder it was fun for me). Not only did the experience of play foster the therapeutic alliance, but research in neuroscience suggests that with repetition our playful interactions may have promoted neuroplasticity by stimulating the creation of new neural patterns (Cozolino, 2010).

Brown (2009) asserts that play is a cornerstone of all personal relationships and that the spontaneous and mutual delight between a child and a parent forms a 'state of play.' Just as parents or caregivers engage in attuned, sensitive and responsive interactions with their child, play therapists demonstrate interest and understanding of the child's emotional world, on a moment-to-moment basis, to build a therapeutic relationship. In doing so, we tap into an evolutionary aspect of our social brain and move forward with the lifelong tasks of building, maintaining and repairing relationships (Badenoch, 2008; Siegel, 2007).

In the context of the play therapy relationship the therapist's use of self is critical to the entire therapy process and must be continually monitored (Yasenik & Gardner, 2012, 2019). Our physical, emotional and verbal use of self all need to be tracked and adjusted in concert with the child's play actions and affective states. To assist a play therapist's understanding of the degree to which they are immersed in the play, and the various ways they make use of the self, the *Degree of Immersion: Therapist use of Self Scale* was developed as part of the play therapy dimensions model (Yasenik & Gardner, 2012). Along with other components of the model, the scale was designed to enhance therapist attunement and strengthen decision making. The scale was recently modified to include the self-system, with an emphasis on embodiment – the degree to which the therapist is aware of their body/energy and internal mental states. When body-mind awareness is on-line, we begin to monitor our internal experiences, in relation to the child, and potentially make better use of our playful self in service of the child's need to re-organise or express troublesome feelings (Yasenik & Gardner, 2019).

During his time at the hospital, much of Bradley's day was focussed on structured activities designed to facilitate speech, motor and physical functioning. While others might have described their activities as 'play', to be effective, research suggests the child's emotional enjoyment in the activity is critical. Gaskill and Perry (2014) also argue that for 'true' play to occur, the child needs to experience joyful pleasure.

Naturally, play activities must be chosen that match the child's development. In the case of Bradley, I used a variety of sensory materials including sand, clay (accessed by digging in his backyard),and messy play with food items he was familiar with, such as pasta. In discussing the EPR developmental paradigm, Jennings (1990, 2014) notes that during the embodiment (E) stage the child's embodied experiences are essential for establishing a 'body-self' and are critical in forming security and trust. Starting at the E stage with play materials and activities Bradley was familiar with, and driven to explore, I likely reduced his anxiety and increased the 'fun factor' (joy).

As our work progressed, I gradually introduced the early pretend play ability of de-centration (a sense of other outside the self). As discussed by Stagnitti (2019), 'other' or doll-related play is indicated when the child imposes meaning on something or someone outside of themselves. As Bradley's family was highly involved in football (soccer in Canada), a football figure was gradually inserted during messy play. Bradley took great pleasure doing silly things with this character. I gave voice to the character's actions and responses, sometimes with words but often with brief vocalisations such as 'yuck' when the character was given mud to eat. Developmentally, this would be viewed as a higher level of play than self-related play (Westby, 1991).

Over time we moved toward more complex play activities, while maintaining focus on Bradley's play skills and my playful use of self (which at the time I simply summed up to equal the 'fun factor'). Cordier and Bundy (2009) suggest that the basic elements of playfulness are best represented as a continuum. For example, the element of motivation can range from intrinsic to extrinsic, and the element of control can range from internal to external. Another element, constraints of reality, speaks to the degree to which the rules of reality can be bent. Framing, the player's abilities to give and read social cues about how to interact with each other, is often observed when a player must convey the message that what they are doing is still 'play' to enable the play frame to continue. Bradley's ability to frame play was highly constricted due to his processing issues. My task was to exaggerate cues and strengthen the frame through voice tone, body posture and my emotionality. Briefly, my immersion in the play was critical to the process.

Empathy

Axline (1947) was the first to underscore empathy as a core helping dimension in the field of play therapy. Since this time, advances in the neurosciences have brought forward evidence that empathy is an essential component of the therapist-client alliance and is strongly predictive of positive outcomes in therapy (Gaskill, 2014). Empathy is a complex neurobiological process, hard wired into our species, which has evolutionary survival value (Decety & Lamm, 2006). The quality of empathic caring impacts the child's self-regulatory capacity, influencing the child's ability to modulate behaviour, express emotions and engage in social relationships (Gaskill, 2014).

Gaskill (2014) notes that empathy subsumes an array of executive processes such as theory of mind, agency and perspective taking. These 'newer' empathic functions, so to speak, are layered on top of phylogenetically 'older' social and emotional capacities. In looking at this structure, Decety (2011) proposed an integrative processing model of empathy that includes both a bottom-up processing of affective sharing and a top-down processing that includes motivation and self-regulation factors. Briefly, the bottom-up processing of the affective aspects of empathy relates to the person's experience of emotion resulting from observation of another's mental state. At this lower brain level, phenomenon associated with the mirror neuron system is present – referred to as emotional contagion or mimicry (Rizzolatti, 2005). The affective aspects of empathy, which develop at a much younger age than the cognitive aspects, are involuntary and rely on mimicry, resulting in a somatosensory resonance between the child and another. This process is largely adaptive and has attachment value for the child. An exception to this occurs when a child is exposed to someone who is overly distraught, at which point the child's regulating capacities become overwhelmed, leading to over arousal and self-focused emotional reactions (Gaskill, 2014). The implication for play therapists is the need to understand and employ strategies that impact lower brain functioning, while in some cases avoiding cognitive strategies that have limited benefit at the lower neurological level (Gaskill, 2014).

At the top level of Decety's integrative model, executive processes are accessed to modulate the emotional experience (top-down processing). Developmental stages have been proposed for empathy and play therapists must recognise there are slow, incremental steps toward empathic competency. Furthermore, we must not only consider the developmental stage of the child, but also their personal histories and unique individual differences (Gaskill, 2014). Play therapists should in fact hold a dual focus on empathy – as a therapeutic tool and as a desirable therapeutic outcome (Gaskill, 2014). Play at the E stage, or sensory-motor level, is believed to contribute to the development of self-capacities that are critical to gains in empathic responding.

Upon reflection, my interactions with Bradley included high levels of empathic attunement to his play actions and fleeting interpersonal behaviours. My intent to express interest, verbally and non-verbally, and convey warmth and sensitivity, created a state of emotional attunement through the neurological coupling of mirror neurons. When combined, these forces contributed to Bradley becoming more connected to the play and deriving joy from our playful interactions. Over time, I noticed fewer pivots or fragmentation in Bradley's play behaviours, relative to when we first began. A significant turning point occurred when Bradley handed me a lump of clay, gesturing that I should throw it to make a 'splat' noise as he had just done. It seems the repetitive sensory play helped Bradley make meaning of external sensory stimuli (that clay could be used for many purposes, including making funny noises). This moment in play also signalled an emergence in Bradley's empathic abilities. Years later, I wish I could have explained to Bradley's mother, and team members, why moments like this count.

Attachment

Attachment, often referred to as an affectional bond, operates across the lifespan and enhances survival because it keeps the infant close to their adult caregiver (Bowlby, 1988). Securely attached children communicate their needs with behaviours and emotional signals, usually making it easier for others to make accurate inferences about what the child needs, physically and psychologically. The caregivers reflective functioning, their ability to reflect on their experience and the experience of their child, is critical to this process. The secure pattern of relationship development in childhood is the pattern most associated with resilience and positive outcomes during school-age years as well as adulthood (Sroufe, 2005; Sroufe & Siegel, 2011).

Belonging, in an attachment sense, means having an 'other' who is available to empathically regulate overwhelming experiences that are part of the child's emerging sense of self (Powell, Cooper, Hoffman, & Marvin, 2014). Through countless experiences of being soothed, comforted and co-regulated or calmed, an internal sense of security and trust evolves (Powell et al., 2014).

In discussing the Circle of Security (COS) intervention, Powell et al. (2014) assert that through the co-regulation of emotions the child learns self-regulation. However, these authors do not view self-regulation as the ultimate goal. Instead, the desired goal is for the child to co-regulate and/or self-regulate, depending on which mode best serves the child in each situation. Within the COS protocol, this balance is partly described as autonomy-within-relatedness and relatedness-within-autonomy. In the play therapy process, just as in the parent-child dance of attunement, the therapist assists in balancing or mediating these two factors. Core play therapy skills such as tracking play actions, restating content and reflecting affect, fundamentally attend to the child on a moment-to-moment basis, particularly when the child is exploring their world and looking for autonomy-within-relatedness. These core play therapy skills and techniques function in much the same way as parental responses to the child's need to 'delight in me as I explore' (the top half of the circle). When in a calm state and the child signals a need for relatedness-within autonomy, they are asking the other to 'delight' in them and show they 'get' their emotions through matching the child's emotional state with tone of voice, facial cues and touch. Stern (1995) speaks of 'feeling-shape' in reference to the intensity, duration, rhythm, contour and quality of a given emotional experience. When a child experiences, or rather feels the adult sharing an emotion, it enhances their connection with both the adult and their own positive internal state. When upset, the child may need (or signal) the caregiver to 'comfort me'. However, the child may also need (or signal) the caregiver to 'organise my feelings' (the bottom half of the circle). At this point the child requires assistance to organise and make sense of an internal experience. Many play therapists will recognise the driven quality of post-traumatic play represents the child's need to make sense and re-organise some part of a traumatic ex-perience. Mastery play also functions in this same realm, whereby the child uses play to make sense and gain mastery over some aspect of their lived experience.

Foundational to the COS protocol is the concept of *being-with* a child as they move around the top and bottom of the circle, using their secure base to support exploration, and being welcomed back to their safe haven. While the experience of sharing a broad range of emotions with an attachment figure promotes security of attachment, being able to experi-ence the full range of emotions without fear of losing coherency, ac-cording to Powell et al. (2014), is critical to an internal sense of security. The concepts of belonging, *being-with*, and holding are readily translated to the play therapy relationship and are embedded in core models of play therapy.

Bradley was a child whose processing issues made the exploration of his world challenging, confusing and, at times, overwhelming. Although he was driven to engage in sensory play and required a range of experiences to fully master the E stage, he needed someone who could both comfort and or-ganise his feelings. I believe I was very responsive and sensitive on the comfort side, as were his parents, but I was slow at picking up on the need to organise his feelings. One day the light bulb came on for me when I observed Bradley's mother introduce a Halloween character of his older brother. Bradley's response to the texture and the noise the character made seemed to be one of surprise, whereas his mother read and responded to his cues as if he was scared. By suggesting that she think of Bradley's behaviour as exploratory and 'curiosity seeking', and his response as one of 'surprise', Bradley's mother started down a different track by trying to help Bradley organise and make sense of his experiences. Over time, this type of orga-nising response likely contributed to a more coherent sense of self. Equally important, Bradley's mother, who needed time to shift her view and re-sponse style, intuitively began to initiate repairs when ruptures occurred in the relationship, particularly when she misread Bradley's requests for or-ganising as a signal of distress. Siegel (2001) suggests that interactive repair is critical to the development of healthy and secure attachment as the adults' effort to repair the relationship helps re-establish an emotional connection fundamental to an attuned relationship. It also communicates to the child that negative emotions can be tolerated and resolved.

Social competence

As children develop they acquire competencies across many domains, including social, emotional, cognitive, linguistic and physical functioning. While social skills refer to discrete learned behaviours for interacting with others and performing specific tasks, social competence is more broadly defined as the individuals' personal and social maturity in multiple domains (Raver & Zigler, 1997). As such, it is imperative that a contextual and developmentally sensitive approach be taken when examining social competence. Commonly identified developmental tasks, such as peer acceptance and compliance with societal rules of conduct, often constitute general domains of competence. However, it is crucial that practitioners understand the distinguishing features of social competence within developmental periods. A discrete and discerning view of social competence not only provides the practitioner with a holistic view of the child, but it can help tailor interventions.

Social competence develops because of interpersonal interactions and is often measured by pro-social behaviours (Howes, 2000) and positive peer relationships (Rose-Kasnor, 1997). An increasing body of research identifies that social skills and peer relationships are a positive indicator of school readiness (Coolahan, Fantuzzo, Mendez, & McDermott, 2000). Correspondingly, children identified as academically at risk are potentially more prone to displaying deficits in social functioning and do less well in school than their socially adjusted peers (Ladd, Kochendorfer, & Coleman, 1997).

Play behaviours provide a window to view development, particularly social development. Developmental theorists such as Piaget (1967), Vygotsky (1976) and Erikson (1968) viewed play as fostering social development and identified children's peer play as a primary context for the acquisition of important social competencies (Fisher, 1992). For example, Piaget (1967) asserted that play was a medium through which children practise social collaboration skills and learn to coordinate multiple points of view (perspective-taking). Through interactions with peers in play, the child moves away from egocentric perspectives, toward acknowledging realities outside of their own views (Fisher, 1992). Briefly, play interactions within the peer group provides feedback fundamental to the socialisation process (Fisher, 1992; Raver & Zigler, 1997). Not surprisingly, research has demonstrated significant correlations among pre-schoolers' levels of socio-dramatic play, measures of social competence, and peer acceptance (Fantuzzo et al., 1995).

Schaefer (2012) notes there are three main types of interactive peer play that foster social skills and positive peer relationships. Rough-and-tumble play is thought to encourage the development and maintenance of relationships, as it affords opportunities to practise appropriate peer interactions while engaging in various social roles (Pelligrini & Perlmutter, 1988; Schaefer, 2012). Socio-dramatic play provides children with opportunities to expand their skill sets by taking on various roles in the context of a social story. A third type, game play, also has a varied and strong impact on the development of social competence. During game play children learn to co-operate, problem solve, take turns and share. Perhaps at a deeper level, game play also affords opportunities for the development of empathy, reciprocity and perspective taking.

Several studies indicate that children with higher levels of pretend play are more competent in social interactions with peers, have greater emotional understanding, make greater use of narrative language and demonstrate narrative competence (Stagnitti, 2009). Pretend play also facilitates convergent and divergent thought, language-literacy, impulse control, perspective taking and socialisation (Westby, 1991). Stagnitti (2019) argues that pretend play, or play scripts reflecting the child's daily life, provide evidence of how the child expresses their growing sense of their autobiographical narrative. This growth is exemplified in the following case of Sammy, where symbolic representation of lived experiences, woven into his play narrative, deepened his sense of self and expanded his range of social competencies.

Case example: Sammy and the three-legged cat

Sammy was referred for play therapy by his parents, upon the recommendation of a child and adolescent psychiatrist. Sammy was a premature baby who spent two months in hospital prior to going home with his parents. Once home, he continued to be tube fed and required medical follow-up for a range of medical issues including feeding, sleep-related difficulties, asthma and seizures. During his pre-school years Sammy was followed by an intensive, multi-disciplinary treatment team. At the point of transitioning to grade one, which triggered the termination of preschool services, Sammy's parents sought additional support for themselves and their six-year-old son.

Upon referral, Sammy's parents reported feeling exhausted. His mother was on an extended work leave due to depression. Sammy's father was actively involved with parenting tasks but expressed feeling overwhelmed and 'bewildered' by Sammy. The father reported that Sammy was a bright but 'lazy' boy who asked adults to do everything for him, including dressing and feeding him. Sammy was also described as an emotionally sensitive and anxious child. The recent death of a pet seemed to trigger worries that his parents may die, or simply leave him. Sammy constantly worried about fires and asked his parents to check their smoke detectors each night before bed. Both parents commented that Sammy struggled immensely with friendships. As his father put it, 'Sammy drives one-way, his way, and watch out if you want to make a left turn and he wants to go right'. At times, Sammy would passively resist or simply ignore his parent's requests; at other times, he would flat out say 'no' or engage in meltdowns marked by screaming, throwing objects and hitting his head. Curiously, Sammy was also a boy who, to coin a term by Ginott (1961), had high levels of 'social hunger'. Sammy desperately wanted to be liked and to have friends. The first time I saw Sammy in my waiting room he had somehow jumped on the lap of another child, who was likely too shocked to say anything, claiming this person was his new 'best friend'.

As noted by Ginott (1961), children with high levels of social hunger are often well-suited to group work. In Sammy's case, he had already been introduced to several small group settings but tended to either disrupt the group or tantrum to avoid going. Sammy also attended at least two structured skill building groups focussing on pragmatic language and social skills. Yes, they also taught children about personal space! While I was reluctant to think Sammy would not benefit at some future point from group work, I believed that therapeutic potency would most occur in the context of an attuned relationship where the therapeutic powers of play, such as empathic engagement, are embedded in a context of playfulness.

For the first few sessions, Sammy consistently brought his stuffie to my office and talked through this character. During brief conversations with Sammy's stuffie, I learned the stuffie had 'exactly' the same feelings as Sammy, only bigger. I explained to the stuffie how we could work together to 'shrink tricky feelings'. I often use this phrase to initially discuss feeling states with young children. In the case of Sammy, whose parents were somewhat alarmed by his anxious tendencies, and quickly moved to comfort rather than organise his feelings, I hoped this phrasing might align us in the same direction. The word 'tricky' was purposefully chosen, as these feelings are neither good nor bad, they are simply tricky and need to be understood (especially when they sneak up on you). Not surprisingly, Sammy commented he would like to help his stuffie. So, our first task was to sort out and organise the stuffie's feelings.

As Sammy was immersed in projective play though his stuffie, I introduced a character called 'Mr. Sneaky'. Using a simple drawing I depicted my Mr. Sneaky, complete with a speaking bubble and the words 'Oh no!' I explained to the stuffie that I had a Mr. Sneaky who tried to outsmart me with tricky thoughts, and that Mr. Sneaky often spoke using the words 'Oh no!' After giving a few examples of what Mr. Sneaky said, such as 'Oh no! I wasn't ready for that!', Sammy's stuffie began giving examples of times when his Mr. Sneaky said things to trick him. Keeping our work at a concrete/visual level, I then asked Sammy if we could make a 'power button' that could help us with ideas to outsmart Mr. Sneaky. We traced each of Sammy's hands. On one hand we drew an outline of Mr. Sneaky; on the other hand, Sammy designed a special power button that could be pushed for an idea to outsmart and 'shrink' Mr. Sneaky.

During consultations with Sammy's parents I emphasised that if we worked to understand Sammy's underlying needs when his tricky feelings surfaced, we could better translate these into 'Oh no!' statements. In turn, this would help construct a power button thought more appropriate to the situation or feeling. Importantly, we weren't necessarily looking for a positive thought to comfort him, such as 'I'm still ok', we were looking for a more powerful thought to organise him. By externalising this process through Mr. Sneaky, the child is also afforded greater distance from their feelings. It wasn't long before Sammy, together with his parents, began to devise plans to outsmart Mr. Sneaky. In a graduated fashion, Sammy helped his stuffie with small situations that were anxiety provoking, such as going downstairs on his own. Several months later Sammy, his stuffie and his parents, flew to visit grandparents, something his parents previously considered impossible.

In the playroom Sammy's play initially appeared fragmented and disorganised. While he enjoyed exploring cars and rescue vehicles, and spoke about building garages, ramps and roads, Sammy's play sequences would typically stop just before the constructional part. I recognised part of the issue was Sammy's difficulty with fine motor skills and motor planning. The other factor was Sammy's reluctance (his parents would say avoidance) to try anything he could not succeed at 100%. Accordingly, Sammy directed me in the construction process and gave stern corrective feedback on minor flaws. I made reflections, through my character, emphasising feelings of uncertainty, frustration and incompetence. Initially, Sammy's response was disapproving. At this point I knew it was critical that I make use of my therapeutic self in a way that would help Sammy tolerate disowned feelings projected on to my character. Through numerous play scenarios and play modalities, including puppets, sandplay and art making, the theme of incompetence continued to surface. However, I noticed Sammy gradually tolerated my errors and, at one point, offered to support me in building a structure. Following this, he even began to offer praise for my efforts, although the burden of construction often rested with my character. Another turning point in the therapy process had occurred. At this moment, I knew empathy for the self was evolving. Over the next several months Sammy engaged in numerous risk-taking activities, inside and outside of our play space. For instance, at school Sammy began to participate in printing and colouring activities.

One day Sammy entered my office at the end of the session with his mother. On my coffee table was a three-legged cat with a bobble head. A funny and rather unusual object recently given to me. Not knowing quite what to do with it, I placed it on my table and forgot about it until Sammy curiously picked it up. Sammy was very intrigued by how the cat, despite only having three legs, could stand. He immediately began to talk about other things the cat could likely do, projecting a sense of 'ability' and competence. We only had a few minutes to explore this object, but Sammy's connection to it was obvious. The next time Sammy returned, I told him a story about the very hungry three-legged cat. Woven into this story was a part about the cat's hunger for friendships, and the rejection he sometimes felt when others didn't understand his unique abilities. Despite having many self-doubts, the three-legged cat tried hard to connect with others and gradually found ways to modify her style by reading and responding to cues from others. This story seemed to be a hit because Sammy immediately wanted to tell his story to the cat, a brave act indicating there was a certain amount of therapeutic potency in my story. As noted by Mills and Crowley (1986), therapeutic potency, accessed through the power of the metaphor, is reflected by changes in how the child thinks or feels about something and, potentially, contains transformative power.

For several weeks, Sammy shared many of his own stories with the three-legged cat. His stories reflected small victories in his daily life, socially and academically. At times, Sammy would even draw a picture about some part of the victory to ensure the three-legged cat understood. Through symbolic re-presentation of his lived experiences, woven into his play narrative, it seemed that Sammy's autobiographical narrative increasingly contained elements of competence and hope. His social appetite remained, but he was now better able to feed himself.

With encouragement Sammy's parents joined the storytelling process, using stories to re-represent or re-play his lived experiences, including Sammy's challenges and victories. From McGilchrist's (2009) perspective, when we reflect to children their experiences, represented in sound, movement, words or symbolic play, we help them with the re-presentation of their bodily experiences. Essentially, the left hemisphere (LH) language processing is returned to the right hemisphere (RH) through metaphor, where the storytelling becomes reconnected to the body for 'meaning making'. If there is sufficient support for the embodied story to become language, the ongoing connection with the other person (listener) fosters development of a natural pathway back to the right hemisphere. The resulting interconnection between hemispheres allows the child to 'make sense' at two levels – in the body and in 'knowing.' The resulting coherence supports interpersonal connection and capacity for attention and self-regulation. According to McGilchrist (2009), each time there is a RH-LH-RH progression, the individual can tell more of their auto-biographical story and, in the process, become more conscious of who they are in the world.

As Sammy's autobiographical memory grew, so did a coherent sense of self. Through the many modalities accessed in Sammy's play therapy process, one could also say that his 'Me' and 'You' maps (Siegel, 2010) became more elaborate, affording greater self-awareness, social perspective and social relatedness.

Conclusion

In each of the four sub-categories of the enhancing social relationships domain we find a complex underpinning of neuro-developmental processes. Explorations of this domain has led us on a journey of self-exploration by examining the therapist's use of self in service of the therapeutic relationship. The critical importance of finding our playful selves has been highlighted, along with the need to be reflective, on a moment-to-moment basis, just as parents do, daily.

References

Axline, V. (1947). *Play therapy*. London, England: Ballantine books.

Bowlby, J. (1988). *A secure base: Parent-child attachment and healthy human development*. London: Basic Books.

Badenoch, B. (2008). *Being a brain-wise therapist: A practical guide to interpersonal neurobiology*. New York, NY: Norton.

Brown, S. (2009). *Play: How it sharpens the mind, opens the imagination, and invigorates the soul*. New York, NY: Bantam Books.

Coolahan, K., Fantuzzo, J., Mendez, J., & McDermott, P. (2000). Preschool peer interactions and readiness to learn: Relationships between classroom peer play and learning behaviors and conduct. *Journal of Educational Psychology, 92* (3), 458–465.

Cordier, R., & Bundy, A. (2009). Children and playfulness. In K. Stagnitti & R. Cooper (Eds.), *Play as therapy: Assessment and therapeutic interventions* (pp. 45–58). London: Jessica Kingsley Publishers.

Cozolino, L. (2010). *The neuroscience of psychotherapy: Healing the social brain* (2nd ed.). New York, NY: Norton.

Decety, J. (2011). Dissecting the neural mechanisms mediating empathy. *Emotion Review, 3*(1), 92–108.

Decety, J., & Lamm, C. (2006). Human empathy through the lens of social neuroscience. *Scientific World Journal, 6*, 1146–1173.

Erikson, E. (1968). *Identity: Youth and crisis*. New York: W. W. Norton & Company.

Fantuzzo, J., Sutton-Smith, B., Coolahan, K. C., Manz, P. H., Canning, S., & Debnam, D. (1995). Assessment of preschool play interaction behaviors in young low-income children: Penn interactive peer play scale. *Early Childhood Research Quarterly, 10*, 105–120.

Fisher, E. F. (1992). The impact of play on development: A meta-analysis. *Play & Culture, 5*, 159–181.

Gaskill, R. (2014). *Empathy*. In A. A. Drewes and C. E. Schaefer (Eds.), *The therapeutic powers of play* (2nd ed., pp. 195–209). New Jersey, Wiley.

Gaskill, R., & Perry, B. D. (2014). The neurobiological power of play: Using the neurosequential model of therapeutics to guide play in the healing process. In C. Malchiodi & D. A. Crenshaw (Eds.), *Play and creative arts therapy for attachment trauma*. New York: Guilford Press.

Ginott, H. (1961). *Group psychotherapy with children*. New York: McGraw-Hill.

Howes, C. (2000). Social-emotional classroom climate in child care, child-teacher relationships and children's second grade peer relations. *Social Development, 38*, 113–132.

Jennings, S. (1990). *Dramatherapy with families, groups and individuals*. London: Jessica Kingsley.

Jennings, S. (2014). Applying an Embodiment-Projection-Role framework in groupwork with children. In E. Prendiville and J. Howard (Eds.), *Play therapy today: Contemporary practice with individuals, groups and carers* (pp. 81–96). London: Routledge.

Ladd, G. W., Kochendorfer, B. J., & Coleman, C. (1997). Classroom peer acceptance, friendship and victimization: Distinct relational systems that contribute uniquely to children's school adjustment. *Child Development, 68*, 1181–1197.

McGilchrist, T. (2009). *The master and the emissary: The divided brain and the making of the Western world.* New Haven, CT: Yale University Press.

Mills, J. C., & Crowley, R. J. (1986). *Therapeutic metaphors for children and the child within.* New York: Brunner/Mazel.

Pelligrini, A. D., & Perlmutter, J. C. (1988). The diagnostic and therapeutic roles of children's rough-and-tumble play. *Children's Health Care, 16*, 162–168.

Piaget, J. (1967). *The child's conception of the world.* London, England: Routledge & Keegan.

Powell, B., Cooper, G., Hoffman, K. & Marvin, B. (2014). *The circle of security intervention: Enhancing attachment in early parent-child relationships.* New York: Guilford Press.

Raver, C. C. & Zigler, E. F. (1997). Social competence: An updated dimension in evaluating Head Start's success. *Early Childhood Research Quarterly, 12*, 363–385.

Rizzolatti, R. (2005). The mirror neuron system and its function in humans. *Anatomy and Embryology, 210*, 419–421.

Rose-Kasnor, L. (1997). The nature of social competence: A theoretical review. *Social Development, 6*, 111–135.

Schaefer, C. E. (2012). *The therapeutic powers of play.* Unpublished manuscript.

Siegel, D. J. (2001). Toward an interpersonal neurobiology of the developing mind: Attachment relationships, 'mindsight,' and neural integration. *Infant Mental Health Journal, 22* (1–2), 67–94.

Siegel, D. J. (2007). *The mindful brain: Reflection and attunement in the cultivation of well-being.* New York, NY: Norton.

Siegel, D. J. (2010). *Mindsight: The new science of personal transformation.* New York: Bantam Books.

Sroufe L. A. (2005). Attachment and development: A prospective, longitudinal from birth to adulthood. *Attachment and Human Development, 7*(4), 349–367.

Sroufe, L. A., & Siegel, D. (2011). The verdict is in. *Psychotherapy Networker, 34–39*, 52–53.

Stagnitti, K. (2009). Children and pretend play. In K. Stagnitti & R. Cooper (Eds.), *Play as therapy: Assessment and therapeutic interventions* (pp. 59–69). London: Jessica Kingsley Publishers.

Stagnitti, K. (2019). Emergence of self through learn to play. In Yasenik, L., and Gardner, K. (Eds.), *Turning points in play therapy and the emergence of self: Applications of the play therapy dimension model* (pp. 43–58). London: Jessica Kingsley Publishers.

Stern, D. (1995). *The motherhood constellation: A unified view of parent-infant psychotherapy.* New York: Basic Books.

Vygotsky, L. (1976). Play and its role in the metal development of the child. In J. Bruner, A. Jolly and K. Sylva (Eds.), *Play, its role in development and evolution.* Harmondsworth: Penguin.

Westby, C. (1991). A scale for assessing children's pretend play. In C. Schaefer, K. Gitlin, & A. Sandrund (Eds.), *Play diagnosis and assessment.* New York: John Wiley & Sons.

Yasenik, L., & Gardner, K. (2012). *Play therapy dimensions model: A decision-making guide for integrative play therapists.* London, UK: Jessica Kingsley Publishers.

Yasenik, L., & Gardner, K. (2019). Turning points and the understanding of the development of self through play therapy. In L. Yasenik, & K. Gardner (Eds.), *Turning points in play therapy and the emergence of self: Applications of the play therapy dimensions model* (pp. 15–42), London, UK: Jessica Kingsley Publishers.

Chapter 12

An hour at Le Mans

Increasing strength and resilience through play

Henry Kronengold

A child's play opens so many windows, both conscious and unconscious, that carry emotional resonance. Important relationships, sense of self, cognitive and affective preoccupations can all manifest in a child's play, while the back and forth of play offers a view of how a child may navigate their interpersonal world. One of many opportunities in play is the utilisation of a child's natural language to enhance their personal strengths via their burgeoning creativity, capacity for problem solving and self-regulation. It is in play that a child is often able to connect to those stronger parts of the self that strengthen the resilience that is critical to a child's ongoing development.

The use of play to enhance personal strengths has a longstanding place in the literature of child development (Lyons-Ruth, 2006), education (Paley, 2004) and child psychotherapy (Schaefer & Drewes, 2014). Psychological factors and functions identified as enhanced by play include creative problem solving, resilience, empathy, social and cognitive development, self-regulation and self-esteem (Schaefer & Drewes, 2014). The mutative power of play has been emphasised using both direct techniques meant to support a child's skills and more indirect approaches that rely primarily on metaphor and relational factors as a means to access a child's capacity to manage their daily world (Crenshaw, Brooks, & Goldstein, 2015; Kronengold, 2017). In this chapter, the role of play in enhancing a child's strengths, particularly in play that is shared, negotiated and embodied, is discussed. This chapter aims to integrate different approaches to play based on a given child's personality style and needs at various moments. As each child, not to mention family, may be unique in presentation, it follows that each child's path of strength and resilience will likewise be distinct.

Six-year-old Danny loved the blocks, Legos and vehicles in my office. He would begin a session excitedly, arranging and planning all sorts of grand designs and adventures. If only he could follow through on one of them. Our first sessions consisted of Danny starting what he was sure would become an architectural masterpiece, light speed spaceship or turbocharged racecar, only for the session to derail moments later as Danny's ability to build, or in his estimation the poor quality of my materials or my assistance, led to frustration, anger and even tears. I had expected this turbulence as Danny presented as an eager, bright and related young boy who greatly struggled to manage disappointment and whose frustrations often led to tantrums at home and struggles at school and with friends. Danny's parents did their best to both accommodate his sensitivities and ignore his outbursts, though, being human, they admittedly lost their cool at times. I was mostly concerned how Danny's frustrations were also getting in the way of his learning and social/emotional development, as Danny's annoyance with an uncooperative wooden block mirrored his difficulty with the necessary stumbles and trials of literacy, while his exuberance and warmth, which had helped him develop friendships, had been eclipsed by an aggressive frustration that was starting to repel his peers. There is also an internal sense of self that can begin to coalesce around frustration, and, unaddressed, it can lead to a darker persona that revolves around a stew of avoiding challenges and expressing upset with any perceived weakness or vulnerability. As he started our fifth session together, Danny took a familiar spot near my toy closet as we proceeded to play.

'Where's the police car?' Danny asked, as he rifled through a bin filled with toy cars. His actions purposeful, I could see Danny had a particular idea in mind as he took out the Hot Wheels racing tracks and grabbed a few cars from the bin. 'I'll take a look', I said, 'I think I left it in the castle'. Danny frowned for a moment, the car in the castle suggested someone else had been playing with the police car and I had seen his rivalrous feelings on display a week earlier when Danny gleefully took apart a Lego structure left behind earlier by another child. It was hard for Danny to feel good enough about his own play, his own creations and his own skills. The insecurity manifested in his annoyance in the same way he struggled with his siblings and his peers. Prior to our session I had listened to a message from his teacher detailing Danny's screaming fit at recess as he joined his friends in a game of baseball before a dropped ball devolved into a mix of anger and tears.

'Hurry up, why didn't you put it back with the rest of the cars?' an annoyed Danny asked, or better said, criticised. I paused a moment so our back and forth would slow down, sensing a chance to work a little on his frustration. 'Ah, I hear the frustration in your voice. I know. It's annoying the car isn't where you want it'. Danny quickly picked up the conversation, 'We need to get going already. How much time do we have left?' I rolled the car over, making a police car sound along the way, as I continued to observe, 'I think we're ok with time, though I know you don't always love it when I say something. Also not so much when someone else has been playing with the toys. Totally get it. It's ok. You're not the only one'. Danny sat quietly for a few seconds and we worked on the tracks together. I had said what I wanted and now it was time to play and let things simmer a bit as Danny worked ambitiously on the tracks. There's a certain skill and planning with these tracks. Mostly they're straight but I have a few curved ones which, when properly placed, offer many possibilities to wind around my office. Then there are the little blue plastic pieces that link one track to another. Crucial to the building, they can also come loose or disconnect, rendering useless even the best laid plans. Not surprisingly, Danny's patience quickly wore thin as the combination of uncooperative blue pieces, lack of sufficient curves and the frustrating presence of walls in my office fed his growing annoyance. I could see Danny's muscles tensing, his teeth starting to grit as he grew increasingly upset.

In play therapy circles, therapists often equate play with creativity and problem solving. But how do we get to this creative place? Is developmental progress always a natural consequence of play? Vygotsky said, 'In play a child always behaves beyond his average age, above his daily behaviour. In play it is as though he were a head taller than himself' (Vygotsky, 1967, p. 16). But is that necessarily true? Was Danny behaving above his age when he played? Did play naturally offer him an opportunity for developmental progress or was it in fact a setup for regression? While this discussion is not meant as a deep exploration of Vygotsky's underlying theories of development, a further look into his ideas about play paints a more complex picture. For Vygotsky, this inherently developmental and powerful notion of play is quite advanced, with an emphasis on imaginative and shared play that relies on a child's capacity to create roles, follow rules and use abstraction (Bodrova & Leong, 2015; Scharer, 2017). For Vygotsky, play is based on the notion that the child has already developed capacities for reflection and self-regulation that allow play to be a forum for enjoyment and growth. Such play is often missing among many children who present with emotional or developmental vulnerabilities. The challenge for therapists is to consider the use of play and the role of the therapist to nurture development in a way that addresses the child's needs and enhances their strengths. I have no doubt that many children will use the naturally creative foundations of play on their own, but others, children such as Danny, require a very particular type of play space, typically with a co-regulating partner, that allows for the growth to occur. Otherwise, Danny would have just grown upset and repeated the same cycle of frustration, vulnerability, anger and likely self-loathing indefinitely. Sometimes, we need a little help to realise what we're actually capable of doing.

'Danny, can you help me with this track. It's driving me nuts'. Yes, I chose words to reconnect to a quickly regressing Danny, but I chose to put the vulnerability and difficulty on myself rather than on Danny. I thought the displacement would be safer and more digestible. He had plenty of experience with people sympathising, empathising and lecturing him regarding problem moments. I knew that Danny basically shut off emotionally as soon as his own weakness was put into the spotlight. There was just too much vulnerability for him to handle. My problems on the other hand could be useful.

'These tracks suck!' Danny exclaimed, but shifted over to help me. 'You may have a point there', I said, 'those blue thingies', I remarked as I gave a shudder before continuing. 'But, I do feel like building something, how about you?' Danny nodded his head up and down. 'Ok, let's try this, shall we?' I suggested, as Danny and I, in fits and starts, worked on the tracks. We worked on keeping the tracks together, especially as they easily separated the longer we built. We'd work on the road and then I'd pause and wonder where to go, giving Danny some space to come up with an idea. We'd try out a segment; maybe even do a few tracks to see how it would work out before completely committing ourselves. As we did the project together, I saw a much calmer version of Danny. A stronger child who had ideas, who could handle twists and turns, literally and figuratively, and perhaps most of all, a child who could be a playmate. After about 15 minutes, Danny and I looked over the office with most satisfied looks on our faces. Before us lay a wonderfully spacious race track with plenty of open road space, several tricky turns, a challenging incline built by layering the tracks over a few blocks, and a tunnel entrance that ran under my sofa. Nodding approvingly at one another, we went back to the car bin to choose our vehicles. I chose a bright yellow race car that I knew was deft at managing the narrow tracks while Danny picked a multicoloured, striped, formula one race car that he deemed the coolest amongst my collection. 'A couple of trial runs?' I suggested but Danny was way ahead of me already, ready to launch his car through the mazy run. 'Mine will get there faster!' he charged, asking me to time the runs. A competitive race would be great and a wonderful opportunity for Danny to practice his regulation, frustration and secure sense of self. My only concern was that he had been ready to toss the tracks out the window about 20 minutes earlier. Perhaps a competitive race was premature. But, before I had a chance to consider an alternative, Danny's car was on the move. At least momentarily.

Danny's car hit a snag trying to head up an incline and rolled backwards. To his credit, Danny was ok, and gave it an extra push before it stopped again midway under the coach. 'Hang on', he said as he ran to crawl under and hit the pretend ignition. 'Ok!' he called out and I gave a thumbs up sign that lasted a few seconds until his car took the next turn poorly and flew off the track. When to intervene and when to let a feeling run its natural course? When do we help a child overcome an obstacle to feel a sense of strength and mastery? When do we refrain from intervening so we don't prevent a child's natural coping from occurring? When do we help a child manage his anxiety and when does a therapist need to figure out how to manage his own nerves so that a child can experience a needed cycle of upset, calm and strength?

I waited to see how Danny would manage this moment. His frustration had been growing as his car stalled and crashed but I'd admired Danny's ability to get this far in our session. We had already gone much further in our play, both in our building, our shared experience and the racing narrative than we had in our prior sessions. I wanted him to see how far he had come but I also didn't want to foreclose on Danny's emotional experience. If his frustration were to emerge more strongly, I also wanted to see its direction at this point. Would Danny turn on himself? Me? The tracks? The cars? Someone or something else?

Danny stomped over to the corner to retrieve his car. His body had tightened again, his face pinkish and heading towards red. Twisting his head in my direction, Danny hurled accusations my way, 'I knew we should have made the turn before! That was your idea! You put it together the wrong way!' As Danny's anger grew I wanted to help contain it. I didn't see the point in him just spewing nor did I want to lock the anger away. I just wanted it to stay in the room without becoming overwhelming. If Danny could manage through the upset, he wouldn't need to fear such disappointments and feelings, and could trust he'd come out the other side. So, I paused, thinking for a second if I wanted to address Danny's accusations directly, through the play or just empathise for a moment.

I had been most pleased at Danny's ability to keep his play going, so, I decided I'd stay in that role and see how things would go. I made a quick engine revving sound and brought my racecar over to the accident scene. 'Whoa', I deepened my voice as an imaginary car; 'I saw the whole thing from over there. You guys ok?' Danny paused for a split second, his face softening ever so slightly as I saw the surprise flicker in his eyes. He had expected a different response, something along the lines of a prolonged negotiation, lecture or some other such drama. He looked at me and then my racecar, then back at his own car who subsequently began speaking in his own deepened voice. 'I was going through that turn but it too was turny', Danny's car explained, his voice more regulated now. 'Yeah', my car nodded, 'I hate those too turny turns, someone's gotta fix those'. I decided to mutter a step further, 'Turny turns', my car added in frustration, hoping that as my car voiced the upset, in the context of our shared play, Danny would be able to handle his feelings and move forward.

Danny looked over the tracks for a moment, seemingly taking in the work of the past 30 minutes or so, and returned to the turn where his car had gone off the rails. He put his car up to his face and began speaking in the car voice, 'I have an idea to fix it', his car intoned, 'get me another straight track and bring over some blocks'. 'Sure thing', my own car replied, as I happily went over to grab the materials, delighted that Danny had weathered the disappointment by using our play and had now gone even deeper into allowing himself to inhabit this streamlined racecar. He directed me to help smooth out the sharp turn and added a couple of blocks to slow it down a bit. I was pleased but Danny was just getting started. 'Ok!' He announced back in his own voice. 'Welcome everyone to the grand prix racing championship! Who are our contestants?' At that, he brought his car back and replied to his own question, 'I am here to win the race!!' Danny continued back in his own voice again, dialoguing with himself, 'OK, we have our first contestant. Is there anyone else here to challenge him?' Taking the invitation, in fairness a bit warily given these ups and downs, I cleared my throat as a bit of a dramatic pre-announcement, brought my own car over, and confidently declared, 'Yes, I am here for the grand prix as well. I am here to win this race!' 'Ok', Danny replied. 'We have two contestants for the grand prix. Get your engines ready'. At this Danny, revved his car at the spot we had begun building our tracks and he told me to do the same with mine. I followed. We had a quick exchange where I wondered how we'd have a race on single lane track but Danny assured me we'd be able to do it. Not entirely convinced, I agreed to give a try. 'Ready!' Danny asked. 'Set!' he called out. 'Go!!!' He bellowed, as our cars took off down the track, with Danny in the lead and my car in hot pursuit.

Managing disappointment and regulating through frustration is one thing, but handling the sense of security and resilience to manage a competition is an entirely different challenge. The ability to deal with one's feelings of aggression, disappointment, anger, anxiety and at times failure is a hard ask, particularly for a child as prone to upset as Danny. I worried at this point about the competition revving up too quickly and of Danny getting close to the close of a session, which had thus far been so groundbreaking for him. I wanted to end this session well, and was concerned that if Danny became upset, he'd mostly remember the negative ending rather than all the positives of our time that day. But, on the other hand, it was his idea to take us into this competitive space, perhaps signaling that we needed to do some work here. Perhaps I needed to trust that even if things went south, Danny would have the resilience to get back into the fray next time. So, I decided I'd split the difference, add some competitive heat and see where things went. I could always titrate the tension, as I kept a close eye on the clock sitting above the underground track passage that Danny and I had built.

'Shifting gears!' I called out, as my car went flying over Danny's and took the lead. Danny didn't miss a beat, 'Not so fast!' he called out as well, 'Gear three – now!' and he flew right back over my car to regain position. 'Hmmm', my car growled, through imaginary car teeth. Around the cars sped as Danny and I made various revving and skidding noises. 'Hyper gear speed!' Danny exclaimed and his car pulled away. I thought again whether I should just leave it. But Danny and I were playing and I wanted to respect this stronger part of him. 'Super hyper-phase speed 100! Go!!' I called out and with this my car went into the super flying phase, leaping over Danny's car. Danny stayed calm, 'Better be careful'. he chimed, as

I looked back at his car for a second. We were headed close to that hairpin turn again and I had a feeling on how to play this one. I pushed my car forward with strength, knowing the likely outcome. Danny smiled for a second to watch.

'Boom!' he narrated, with a crashing sound. My car had picked up too much speed heading to the turn, flying off the track, ricocheting off my castle, and spinning upside down on the floor. I surveyed the wreckage. 'Oh man, that kinda hurt', as my car exhaled. 'Yeah', Danny remarked as he slowed a bit to talk to my car, 'The hyper thing, what's it called again?' Danny asked. 'Super hyper-phase speed 100', I intoned seriously. 'Yeah, super hyper-phase 100 was too fast. You flew over the turn. Sorry. Here, I'll tow you in'.

I have to admit I wasn't expecting help. I had wondered if Danny would delight in his triumph, perhaps tease me for crashing or at the very least just ignore my car as he focused on his victory. He did none of those, though I'm sure he was happy to win the grand prix. But, instead, our play had allowed Danny to stop for a moment, trusting his speed, his car a stand-in for himself, and offered the sense of strength that in turn can foster a degree of empathy for someone else. He called in the police car from early in our session to help out sort out my car, pretended to connect my wreck to the back of the police, and calmly finished out the race, crossing the finish line as he directed me to help have the other cars cheer the winning moment. He even styled himself a victory lap. I respected his style points.

I looked over at the clock and our time was basically done. I brought my car up again, 'Well run race my friend. Congratulations on your victory and thanks for helping me out there. Appreciate it', I said in my most no-nonsense racecar gladiator voice. I returned to my regular voice and spoke now as myself. 'That was quite the race. We are going to have to say goodbye for today'. 'Wait', Danny replied, 'Do you have those magnets. I'll do it fast', he added in a half-demanding half-questioning tone. The magnets, yes, those little things on my desk from when I tried to fix a faulty door. Danny and I had talked about those in our first session when he looked over everything in the office. Not a bad memory, I thought to myself and I reached for a magnet and handed it over. 'Thank you ladies and gentlemen, now for the awards ceremony!' Danny began as I motioned with my hand to speed it up a little as I did have someone waiting for me. Danny nodded. 'The winner of the grand prix 2015! Hurray for the blue, red and yellow striped supercar!!!' As Danny had the cars cheer, I applauded, and then stuck a small circular magnet on the car as a medal. 'Well deserved', I said. 'That car went through a lot. A very impressive victory'. I paused a second before continuing. 'We gotta go. Can you help me put these away?' So, Danny and I tossed the tracks and cars quickly in their bins. 'Can I put the car on the side with the medal', Danny asked. 'Sure, you know the deal though right?' 'Yes', he answered. 'If it stays it stays, but if someone wants to play with it they can'. Impressed, I nodded, put the prizewinner on my bookshelf and Danny and I said goodbye for the day.

Danny's difficulties with frustration, upset and anger were not going to end that day. Challenges with self-regulation, mastery, confidence and resilience don't disappear in an hour. A child's sense of self, based on a feeling of security, mastery, efficacy and relatedness is not built in an hour at an imaginary racetrack. A week later, Danny was angry at me once again, this time for having wooden blocks that were too smooth and therefore kept falling down during building. But, that said, a glimpse of Danny's capabilities and strengths, for both of us, offered a foundation of change moving forward. I trusted that Danny would be able to build on our session, using play that was created, sustained and shared. I trusted in his capacity to strengthen his ability to regulate and manage emotions, to negotiate difficult moments and to tap into his obvious intelligence and creativity. Perhaps most of all, I trusted that our enjoyment in this session, our sense of fun that is so fundamental to play, would continue to build via our relationship, and, in turn, Danny would develop outside relationships with peers and teachers as he made steady progress with respect to his academic, social and emotional development. My work with Danny, our scenes on the racetrack, relied on play as an engine for Danny's growth in a range of psychological, social and emotional venues.

In this way, Danny's burgeoning play could serve as a springboard for experiences outside of my office, where Danny would be able to consolidate his growing strengths across social, emotional, and cognitive realms. Danny's growing use of imaginary play, growing alongside his capacity to self-regulate, tolerate frustration, and enjoy our relationship, would allow for the crucial real-world experiences that would further enhance his self-esteem, his capacity for empathy and his overall development.

Of course, our sessions nonetheless raise questions in mind as I think about how best to nurture a child's developmental strengths and progress. I chose to inhabit my characters and imbue them with emotion that allowed for an emotionally charged experience in therapy. While I was certainly looking to titrate the amount of affect in the room, it is fair to wonder how our sessions would have played out if I had chosen a more neutral role. What if I hadn't been competitive with Danny? Would our sessions have lacked a necessary emotional edge that allowed him to integrate and work through his capacity for resilience? Perhaps a very accepting and more reflective stance would have helped Danny feel safe and secure in exploring his feelings and been more helpful to him in developing his strengths? How far do we allow a child to experience upset in our work? Again, I looked to allow for some frustration but didn't want Danny's anger or upset to go too far. I was looking to find a place that proved challenging but not overwhelming. But how do we decide on the boundaries of what is useful and not useful in terms of a child's emotional experience in our sessions? How do we know if we're in fact supporting a child's capacity for resilience or shutting down a necessary emotional reaction that helps a child feel understood and known? From a completely different perspective, I also wonder about the place of direct work in enhancing a child's strengths. What is the role of direct strategies in working with frustration tolerance and angry feelings? In these sessions I chose to use play as a dramatic canvas to explore, experience and shift the emotional tempo in ways that I felt fit with Danny's presentation and interests. I emphasised the development of Danny's imaginary play, channeling Vygotsky's notions that such play would serve to further a variety of Danny's developmental skills. But, what about the place of clear skill-building, such as cognitive-behavioural or mindfulness techniques, which can certainly utilise play, to help a child develop these same capacities? Perhaps a child's capacity for imaginary play can in turn be enhanced by directly targeting that child's skills as they relate to basic developmental functions such as self-regulation, self-esteem and resilience.

References

Bodrova, E., & Leong, D. J. (2015). Vygotskian and post-Vygotskian views on children's play, *American Journal of Play*, 7, 371–388.

Crenshaw, D. A., Brooks, R., & Goldstein, S. (Eds.), (2015). *Play therapy interventions to enhance resilience*. New York: Guilford Press.

Kronengold, H. (2017). *Stories from child and adolescent psychotherapy: A curious space*. New York: Routledge.

Lyons-Ruth, K. (2006). Play, precariousness, and the negotiation of shared meaning: A developmental research perspective on child psychotherapy, *Journal of Infant, Child, and Adolescent Psychotherapy*, 5, 142–159.

Paley, V. G. (2004). *A child's work: The importance of fantasy play*. Chicago: University of Chicago Press.

Schaefer, C. E. & Drewes, A. A. (Eds.). (2014). *The therapeutic powers of play: 20 core agents of change* (2nd ed.). New York: Wiley.

Scharer, J. H. (2017). Supporting young children's learning in a dramatic play environment. *Journal of Childhood Studies*, 42, 62–69.

Vygotsky, L. S. (1967). Play and its role in the mental development of the child. *Soviet Psychology*, 5, 6–18.

Conclusion

Athena A. Drewes

Charles Schaefer, who passed away in September 2020, laid the foundation for the field of play therapy nationally and internationally. He left a rich legacy of writings, edited and co-edited books and formed the Association for Play Therapy and the annual International Play Therapy Study Group, which became a think tank of invited play therapy clinicians from around the world. He stressed that play was not just a medium or context for applying other interventions, but that inherent in play behaviours are a broad spectrum of active forces that produce behaviour change. That the basic purpose of psychotherapy is to bring about change for the client. That there are therapeutic factors which are the actual mechanisms that effect change in clients. They are the enzymes that aid in digestion of unresolved material and overwhelming emotions in clients. And, indeed, the therapeutic powers of play constitute play therapy's innermost core, its essence, its 'heart and soul'. They represent a middle level of abstraction between general theories and concrete techniques. Therapeutic powers of play transcend culture, language, age and gender (Schaefer & Drewes, 2014).

Dr. Schaefer (1993) initially presented a list of active ingredients in play that produce a therapeutic change, which included self-expression, relationship enhancement, abreaction and attachment formation. He stressed that a greater understanding of the active forces of change in child and play therapy would not only broaden clinicians' repertoire of treatment strategies but would also aid their ability to tailor them to meet the needs of their individual clients (a prescriptive approach). Dr. Schaefer further believed that, through a better understanding of these change agents, practitioners could become better clinicians, as well as researchers. His list of therapeutic powers of play expanded to 20 core agents of change, and these have become the springboard for this volume (Schaefer & Drewes, 2014).

The therapeutic powers of play transcend particular models of play therapy by defining treatment in terms of cross-cutting principles of therapeutic change. A transtheoretical model of play therapy that helps the play therapist avoid becoming locked into a single theory that they then must apply to all clients in a 'one-size-fits-all' manner. Thus, in using a trans-theoretical play therapy model the clinician selects and adds to their repertoire the best change agents from among all the major theories of play therapy creating a prescriptive and integrative play therapy approach. Theoretical integration, therefore, involves the synthesis of two or more change agents in the belief that the resulting integration will surpass the effect of a single change mechanism (Drewes & Schaefer, 2014). As readers, we get to see this in action in this innovative volume.

The editors of *Clinical Applications of the Therapeutic Powers of Play: Case Studies in Child and Adolescent Psychotherapy* explore the scope and scale of how play can enhance and facilitate therapeutic change in clinical practice. They take the integration of the therapeutic powers of play and case studies to a new level. They have succeeded in accomplishing their goals of filling a gap in the play therapy literature by uniting the therapeutic powers of play with actual case studies, theoretical models and linking abstract theory with practice-based knowledge. This unique volume utilises a transtheoretical approach by bringing in and blending the therapeutic powers of play with several different theories. The theories tapped include the theoretical frameworks of child-centred play therapy, trauma theory, attachment theory and child development. It also blends the therapeutic powers of play with various useful models such as Jennings' embodiment-projection-role (EPR) model, the integrating, theory, evidence and action (ITEA) model of Hitch, Pepin and Stagnitti, the play therapy dimensions model by Yasenik and Gardner and Stagnitti's learn to play program.

Prendiville and Parson open up this comprehensive volume with their Forward. It introduces us to the therapeutic powers of play along with Jennings' EPR model, which supports the child's development of physical, emotional and social identity. They begin by helping us to contextualise the process of therapy in action.

Section 1 sets the scene and landscape of the who, what, why, when and where the powers of play therapy are most effective. Chapters 1–4 give us a lens to track change and focusses in on the traditional play therapy settings that help to address development and sensory play in practice and outdoors in nature. Case examples in these chapters show us how early childhood trauma has stifled developmental, emotional and relational growth. The authors allow us the privilege of seeing how pretend play and therapeutic processing of unresolved material can change the tone of past memories, allowing for the transfer of previously intrusive memories to fade into past memories, and strengthen resiliency.

Section 2 allows us to travel through the continents of sensory, projective, pretense and role play in Chapters 5–8. The authors gracefully weave various theories and models which can soothe and stimulate neurological integration, enhance attachment and address developmental delays. We get to see in action how Jennings' embodiment category is utilised in sensory play, Stagnitti's learn to play model uses small world play to negotiate meaning out of functional play and how role play addresses attachment and offers non-verbal means to heal relational breaks. Role play, projective play, the art and science of pretense play and embodiment play are highlighted in a neuro-sequential approach to healing early life developmental trauma. The book comes alive in the emergence of an integrative framework whereby the 20 therapeutic agents of change are activated and the links between theory and practice emerge.

Section 3, with the final Chapters 9–12, brings most clearly into light all 20 of the therapeutic powers of play and their treatment impact as it integrates further with child-centred play therapy, attachment theory and the play therapy dimensions model by Yasenik and Gardner. This section continues to enrich our understanding of the therapeutic powers with cogent and engaging clinical cases illustrating how play facilitates communication, fosters emotional wellness and resilience, increases personal strengths and enhances social and attachment relations.

Going forward play therapists need to continue to conduct research that will allow for further validation of the powers of play as a change agent both as therapy and within therapy. University play therapy courses need to include and highlight the importance of how play and its therapeutic powers can evoke therapeutic and life-long change. Universities further need to teach an integrated, transtheoretical approach to treatment that advocates clinicians utilising a prescriptive approach so that clients obtain the best and most effective treatment. Dialogue needs to be ongoing to bring awareness of how important play is in the lives of children, and actually for all ages across the spectrum, in healing past wounds and integrating social, emotional, developmental and intellectual spheres.

The beauty of this volume is that it takes the initial steps in reinforcing and bringing alive the value and use of play as an enzyme that aids in the digestion of unresolved material and overwhelming emotions. Through each case example by international authors, we clearly see how the therapeutic powers of play transcend culture, language, age and gender. We are enriched in our learning and practice with the abundance of research presented, the demonstration of the art and science of play and play therapy and most importantly in the weaving of transtheoretical theory with practice, illuminated by the abundance of rich, detailed case studies that highlight and bring alive the therapeutic powers of play! We are indeed indebted to the chapter authors and editors for this visionary step. Eileen and Judi have done a wonderful job with this edition, and it is certainly an added testimony to the enduring legacy of Dr. Schaefer. He was very passionate about the therapeutic powers of play and the need to instill this teaching in play therapists and clinicians. This book certainly helps to pay homage to a great man.

References

Drewes, A. A. & Schaefer, C. E. (2014). Introduction. How play therapy causes therapeutic change. In C. E. Schaefer & A. A. Drewes (Eds.), *The therapeutic powers of play: 20 core agents of change* (pp. 1–7). Hoboken, NJ: John Wiley.

Schaefer, C. E. (1993). *The therapeutic powers of play*. NY: Jason Aronson.

Schaefer, C. E. & Drewes, A. A. (2014). *The therapeutic powers of play: 20 core agents of change*. (2nd ed.). Hoboken, NJ: John Wiley.

Index

Note: *Italicized* page numbers refer to figures, **bold** page numbers refer to tables.

For Product Safety Concerns and Information please contact our EU
representative GPSR@taylorandfrancis.com
Taylor & Francis Verlag GmbH, Kaufingerstraße 24, 80331 München, Germany